UNDERSTANDING YOUR PER

With Myers-Briggs and m

PATRICIA HEDGES discovered her interest in personality when studying with Dr Frank Lake, and later developed this through using the work of Professor David Keirsey. She runs a personal consultancy for groups and individuals, and has lectured on type and temperament in venues ranging from church halls to the QE2. Patricia gives conference weekends to help people understand and make the most of their type and temperament.

Overcoming Common Problems

UNDERSTANDING YOUR PERSONALITY
With Myers-Briggs and more

Patricia Hedges

sheldon**PRESS**

First published in Great Britain in 1993
Sheldon Press, SPCK, Marylebone Road, London NW1 4DU

Third impression 1997

I would like to thank Darley Anderson and Kay Albrecht for all their help.

British Library Cataloguing-in-Publication Data

A catalogue record for this book is available from the British Library

ISBN 0–85969–670–7

Photoset by Deltatype Ltd, Ellesmere Port, Cheshire
Printed and bound in Great Britain by
Biddles Ltd, Guildford and King's Lynn

For Tom, my ISFJ husband

Whatever the circumstances of your life, whatever your personal ties, work and responsibilities, the understanding of type can make your perceptions clearer, your judgements sounder, and your life closer to your heart's desire.

Isabel Briggs Myers
Gifts Differing

Contents

Introduction

How many times a day do you feel confused by the reactions of those around you? How often do you wish you could have some grasp of the ways in which people feel, and think and act?

As we all live and work with each other we are inevitably fascinated, intrigued and also made desperate by the difference and chemistry of our personalities. Most of us have moments when even our own reactions surprise us, especially when we find these are totally at odds with those around us. If only we could bring some understanding of ourselves and everyone else to our everyday relations with people then perhaps life would be smoother and less perplexing!

The aim of this book is to illustrate how different patterns feature in the way we *all* feel, think and act, and also how these patterns can account for many of our misunderstandings in our dealings with people. In the ensuing chapters, you will learn about your own patterns and those of other people in some detail, and how you can benefit by making use of this in your home, work and social life.

Patricia Hedges
1993

1

An Introduction to Type

For thousands of years people have been aware that there are marked differences in human behaviour. As early as 450 BC Hippocrates was suggesting that it was possible to observe four distinct temperaments, and throughout the centuries many other people have supported this theory. But it was the publication of Carl Jung's book *Psychological Types* in 1920 which provided something more tangible. The Swiss physician's work demonstrated that each of us has specific and identifiable characteristics. Though only a small part of his life's work, Jung's book provided a solid base for years of further research.

Among the people who recognized Jung's work on personality as valuable was an American, Katharine Myers, who found that his book confirmed her own ideas. She had already become fascinated and absorbed by observing the differences in those around her, and Jung's theories encouraged and stimulated her to continue working.

Katharine's daughter, Isabel, grew up to share her mother's fascination and commitment to these concepts, and the two women, who were not psychologists, devoted the rest of their lives to researching into Jung's theories. Their painstaking and diligent research carried on for 40 years, in spite of encountering much opposition and finding very little encouragement. At the end of this time, in 1962, they formulated a questionnaire which was able to sort and identify 16 different personality types. This was called the Myers-Briggs Type Indicator (MBTI®), and with this questionnaire they made available the results of their years of research.

At first there was not much enthusiasm for their work, but in 1972 the Center for the Application of Psychological Type (CAPT) was established in Florida as an official research centre. The Center started to collect information and data about personality types, and has now become the world's centre for data about Type.

In 1975 the Myers-Briggs Type Indicator was finally published in the USA by the Consulting Psychologists Press, and continues to be published by them today. It was not long before the Indicator gained recognition, and interest in the information surrounding the MBTI grew rapidly in the 1980s. The research around the MBTI was so solid and meticulous that many people from all over the world have been able to add to this, as it has been found that Type transcends culture.

In recent years the person who has probably contributed most to

® MBTI and Myers Briggs Type Indicator are registered trademarks of Consulting Psychologists Press, Inc.

further research is an American Professor, David Keirsey. He has followed his own line of investigation for nearly 40 years, and his temperament theory is immensely helpful to those of us who find 16 Types rather too many to carry in our heads. Keirseian Temperament theory tells us that the 16 Types divide into four basic Temperaments, and he provides precise and accurate details which let us know how we can recognize these. A number of sections in this book refer to Temperament, and these sections are based on the work of Professor David Keirsey.

It is over ten years since I came to an awareness and understanding of Type. This has brought immense enrichment to my life, made it better balanced and helped me channel my abilities in the right direction. It can do this for you, too, whoever you are and whatever you do.

2
Becoming Aware of
Our Differences

This chapter looks at some of the ways we see different patterns in our lives. The following examples will highlight how you may feel more comfortable with one person's attitude than with another's. See if this is true for you. You can read about these in more detail in Chapter 3.

Tom and Jennifer are different in their needs for sociability. Tom works in an office and spends a lot of his day with other people. He needs time on his own to recharge his batteries, as being with other people for long periods drains him. He is looking forward to a number of quiet evenings at home. Jennifer is different. Her energy is renewed by interaction with other people, and too much time by herself depresses her. So, when she says: 'I'd like to have a few people in to supper this week. I feel I haven't seen anyone to talk to for ages', Tom is amazed; how can Jennifer feel she hasn't anyone to talk to? 'How on earth can you feel like that?' he exclaims. 'Why, only last week John and Susan came to supper!'.

Do you feel more comfortable with Tom's need for more privacy or Jennifer's need for more external interaction?

Derek and Jean, two managers, are employed by a firm of engineering consultants. They meet in Jean's office early one afternoon just before they interview Bob Smith, who is shortlisted for a consultancy job in the company.

Jean feels that the most important things to find out are further details of Bob's background qualifications and the specific experience he has had in the past, and where he has had that experience.

Derek, on the other hand, feels that it is very much more important to find out what ideas Bob can put forward about the job and to look at his potential, in other words to get a view of what he is capable of doing in the future.

As they discuss their interview plans, Jean and Derek's conflicting views become very apparent. Jean is not pleased. She interviews regularly for the company and always bases her decisions on a

3

person's past experience. She likes to question candidates about their background, finding out as many practical details as she can. But Derek also interviews regularly, although he and Jean have interviewed separately until now. He takes a different attitude, as he believes the past is past and that it is the future which really matters. He has a more conceptual mind and expects a candidate to be in a position to put forward suggestions and ideas for their job.

Do you feel more comfortable with Jean's emphasis on facts and past experience, or with Derek's emphasis on future potential?

Carol and Margaret met at a fitness club three months ago and have become good friends. Carol values Margaret's clear and logical mind, and Margaret enjoys Carol's kind and gentle manner. They sometimes meet at weekends, and this Saturday morning are shopping together when Carol says: 'I'm free this afternoon, so I'm going to visit Jane'. Margaret is astounded. She knows Jane slightly and finds her a tiring person to be with; she also knows that Carol has had an exhausting week at work. Margaret replies: 'But you know you're exhausted, why on earth are you going to visit her today?' 'Jane's not got many friends', explains Carol, 'and I feel sorry for her since she broke up with her boyfriend. Anyway, she appreciates me going so much and that always makes me feel good.' Margaret says nothing, but thinks: 'What ridiculous reasons for deciding to visit anyone!'

Carol and Margaret are looking at the situation from different viewpoints. Carol feels it is important to consider how Jane feels towards her, and how her visit might increase harmony between them. As Jane has broken up with her boyfriend Carol feels considerable sympathy towards her. Margaret thinks it is more important to consider things logically and rationally, and since Carol is already tired Margaret feels it is illogical and senseless to make herself more tired by visiting Jane.

Do you feel more comfortable with Carol's more personal way of deciding, or with Margaret's more objective view?

It is Friday evening in the Jacksons' living room. Andrew Jackson is home from work, and he and his wife, Barbara, have just finished their evening meal. Barbara reminds him that his mother is recovering from a minor operation and he should phone her. Andrew says, 'Yes, I will', but during the evening he makes no effort to do this.

Throughout the weekend Barbara keeps reminding him to phone, but it is late Sunday evening before Andrew gets round to it. This annoys her intensely, as the phone call has been on her mind all the weekend. 'If I was phoning *my* mother,' she thinks, 'I would phone on the Friday evening, as I would feel better once I had made the call.' She would much prefer Andrew to do the same and get the call out of the way. Then they could have forgotten all about it.

Andrew fully intended to phone his mother, but he could see no urgency for this. Saturday morning he decides to spend at the squash club, and when he comes home he remembers that two of their kitchen cupboards need repairing, so he spends the remainder of the weekend doing these. Andrew prefers to decide things as he goes along and dislikes life to be too structured and organized. He cannot think why Barbara keeps nagging him all weekend. On Sunday evening he phones his mother.

Do you feel more comfortable with Barbara's need to be more organized and to get things finished, or with Andrew's need to be more open-ended and see what happens?

Conflicts and differences like these happen to us all the time, but it is only when we come to some understanding and clarification of these differences that we start to gain insight. First, we can begin to recognize and identify the different characteristics in ourselves and also in those around us; second, we can come to realize that behaviour which appears to be inconsistent and haphazard does, in fact, have some underlying logic and order to it.

As this book unravels some of the complexities of personality, it will show you how you can identify your own most positive characteristics, and bring to light your best qualities. This will make you feel good about yourself, and help you locate within yourself what it is you should aim for in your life. You will also come to see why some things come easily to you whereas others are very much more difficult.

3

Fundamental Aspects of
Our Personality

This chapter introduces the basic characteristics of personality. The ones which are better developed in us give us our personality type. The personality characteristics we prefer to use are our strongest ones and these are referred to as our *preferences*. It is not that we cannot use our less developed characteristics, rather, it is that we work and live better using our preferred characteristics. These characteristics refer to different aspects (or *functions*) of our interaction with the world.

When we prefer something we like it better than something else. We can only prefer something when we have a choice. So it is with our personality characteristics. We have a choice from four pairs of characteristics, and out of each pair, we choose one, preferred, characteristic. It is then these four preferred characteristics (or Preferences) which make up our personality type (or Type).

As you read about the four pairs of characteristics you will probably find that you feel more comfortable with one characteristic than another. As you then go on to read about these in more detail, you will begin to see the ways in which they relate to your life.

The basic pairs of personality characteristics are as follows:

Extraversion (E) and Introversion (I) These relate to our preference for the outer world or the inner world.

Sensing (S) and INtuition (N) These relate to how we take in information about the world around us.

Thinking (T) and Feeling (F) These relate to the process by which we come to our decisions.

Judging (J) and Perceiving (P) These relate to our preference for a more organized or a more flexible lifestyle.

If you would like to do the Personality Discovery Questionnaire which I have devised you can find details about this in Further Information on page 148. You can then see, as you read on, if you agree with what you said about yourself in the questionnaire.

Extraversion and introversion

Extraversion (E) and Introversion (I) tell us about our *attitude* to the world – whether we have a preference for the outer world of people and things or for the inner world of thoughts and contemplation. Whichever is our preference this is where we get our energy.

Extraverts (Es) and Introverts (Is) need different environments in order to stimulate and re-energize themselves. Extraverts need interaction with other people; they talk and express themselves easily and are outgoing rather than reserved. Introverts need privacy, placing value on time to reflect and consider, and are more reserved than outgoing.

Extraverts are drawn outwards by the needs and demands of the world, whereas Is are drawn inwards by these demands. Where Es are sociable and outwardly friendly – needing to talk out their ideas and lives with others – Is are more separate and detached, needing time on their own to be quiet.

Extravert types need to be in touch with other people – communicating, talking, putting things into action. Their attention is on the outside world. Extraverts make decisions quickly and act on them, dealing with problems on the spot. If they are surrounded by Is at home or at work they find this disturbing, and get impatient as they need feedback and communication from others.

Introvert types are different: they need time apart from other people; this is when they think through problems carefully. They are likely to be slower to do things than Es, preferring to reflect and consider before acting. They tend to be more patient, and their attention is directed inwardly. If they are surrounded by Es at home or at work they tend to find this energy-draining. Sometimes they bottle up their emotions.

We can see that the Extravert's *ATTITUDE* is outward whereas the Introvert's is inward. The statements below relate to each Attitude; see which column you feel most comfortable with.

Extravert Attitude	Introvert Attitude
Enjoy working with people and can be lonely without them. Like to spend quite a lot of leisure time with people too	Enjoy being with people some of the time, but need space for more solitary activities. Need time alone to read, meditate or be quiet
Enjoy being in a group of people, and are generally	Prefer meeting people in small numbers and are better at

7

talkative and friendly. Can feel drained by long period alone	relating to people one at a time; too many people are exhausting and energy draining
Like to hear everyone's news, and interest goes wide and outward	Tend to wait until receive other people's news. More interested in inward reflection
Usually outspoken and make friends easily, know a lot of people	Reserved and may not speak out easily. Make friends slowly but value them
Energy obtained from interaction with others. Can use up energy easily and get exhausted	Renewed from inner resources, and likely to conserve energy rather than expend it
Likely to speak out when with others and to express feeling. Usually talk easily on the phone	When with others need time to think before offering opinions. If others are talking tend not to get a chance. May not speak easily on the phone
Impulsive; think about things after the event	Like to think before acting; on occasions may not act in time
Talk easily about themselves and their views. If surrounded by introverts can find this uncomfortable, as uneasy with silence	Harder to get to know as the best of person is hidden. Find being surrounded by garrulous extroverts painful
More balanced when some introversion is developed	More balanced when some extraversion is developed

According to figures from the USA, extraversion occurs in 70–75 per cent of the general population, and introversion in 25–30 per cent. Also, we can expect to find Es and Is equally among males as females.

Since the Extraverts are much greater in number than the Introverts we can see that Es find it easier to live in the world around them. Introverts are in the minority, and frequently feel pressurized by Es to be more outgoing and sociable. Because Is are smaller in number, and are therefore a minority group, they are sometimes regarded as eccentric and unsociable. We need to value Es and Is equally, as both bring contributions to society but in different ways.

Extraverts often speak more quickly and loudly than Introverts, sometimes using their hands to express what they mean. Introverts tend to speak slower, possibly more quietly, using less facial and body expression.

Extraverts' thoughts and ideas become clear to them as they talk about these to other people; Introverts' thoughts and ideas become clear when they are able to think on their own.

Strong Extraverts, if left on their own too long, become unsettled, needing communication with people. Recharged by this, they can continue to work on their own for a while. Strong Introverts, however, when obliged to be with people for too long, become depleted and exhausted and need to withdraw. Recharged by this, they may be sociable again.

In the home, Es and Is may have difficulty in living together, both needing just what the other cannot give them! The E's need to talk about everything s/he is involved in uses up the I's energy; and if the E has no response from the I, the E redoubles her/his effort to talk even more! Conversely, the I's need for personal space is seldom allowed for by the E. And to protect his/her personal space, the I withdraws further, causing the E to press even more for sociability.

Meetings and get-togethers, whatever they relate to, are usually made up of both Es and Is. Most of us are involved with meetings or groups of one sort or another, whether they are business, social or just groups of friends. Here are some examples of what happens with the E/I preferences.

In a group which has a mixture of Es and Is, it is probably the Es who speak out first, getting their opinions heard. Other Es then continue, and often the Is get left out. This is not intentional: the Es feel that the Is would surely speak if they wanted to. But many Is need peace and quiet to reflect *before* they can speak. And at most groups and meetings such an opportunity does not arise. If there are decisions to be made we get the best from Is if we allow them time to quietly consider the points raised, and then ask for their thoughts.

When we meet Is we need to be aware that the best of them is inside, and in everyday communications we do not meet this. Only when Is know us well, or have built up trust in us, do they show us the best of themselves. This is an important feature of understanding Is, and is covered in more detail in Chapter 11.

But all Is, in order to manage in the world, have developed an extroverted side – though some more than others. If it is necessary for an I to speak out to achieve something they feel is important they will usually do this. They know they are acknowledging the outer world, and they quickly return to their inner world once their task is accomplished.

Many couples have different E and I preferences – being attracted to each other's opposite way of being. Extraverts are drawn to Is' quiet strength, and feel they provide a balance to their own liveliness. Introverts are drawn to Es' openness and friendly manner. Living together, however, is another experience, and both come up against a different Attitude to living. Understanding a partner's attitude can help both to get along better.

Sensing and iNtuition

Sensing and iNtuition tell us how we become aware of the world around us, and how we take in information. They tell us how we notice people, things and situations, and what we are likely to absorb from what we read and what people say to us. These are, perhaps, the most important preferences to understand about ourselves. Our subsequent decisions and how we carry these out depend on the way in which we perceive or notice things. This is why we call Sensing (S) and iNtuition (N) our Perceiving functions.

Our Sensing qualities take in information through our five senses – sight, hearing, touch, taste and smell. If your preferred way of functioning is through Sensing you are likely to place importance on the specific and the particular; you tackle things one step at a time, live in the present, read and follow instructions, and are literal-minded, placing importance on facts; you are probably realistic and prefer the actual to the possible, choosing to do something rather than speculating about it.

The Sensing (S) person is generally grounded in present day realities, likes things that are definite and measurable and handles practical matters well. Problems are approached systematically, step-by-step, with patience for precise factual work. Sensing people often absorb facts, even if they do not need them. They enjoy using skills they have already learnt, and do things methodically, concentrating on the present. They may, therefore, be less aware of the consequences for the future.

INtuitive people function quite differently: they take in and perceive information in a more wide-ranging and broader way, absorbing the data as a whole rather than in separate parts. If your iNtuitive function is dominant you may skip facts and directions, tackling projects and work in your own way. Sometimes you have your head in the clouds, being more interested in ideas and possibilities than present day realities, and you may be thinking about what might happen in the future. You enjoy learning new skills rather than continually practising old ones.

The iNtuitive tends to live in the future, always seeing new possibilities and ways of changing and improving things. She or he feels that the present situation can be made better and enjoys thinking out ways of doing this. Sometimes the N is unaware of present-day realities, such as where keys, ticket or wallet have been left. INtuitives look at the whole picture rather than the details, and can see patterns and relationships between people and things. New projects are exciting to them as they can get their teeth into them, and they often work by hunch. Information is not taken in in a meaningless way, as everything taken in is linked and connected.

Here are some statements which relate to our Sensing and iNtuitive functions, letting us know how we Perceive the world around us. One of these will be dominant for you, which is it?

Sensing function	INtuiting function
Realistic, practical and sensible	More imaginative and reflective
Follows instructions; notices details	May ignore instructions; jumps in impulsively; oblivious of details
Literally-minded; uses established methods	Inventive; likes change and variety
Believes the past is important and that we should make our decisions on past experience	Believes the future is important and that we should base our decisions on future possibilities
Deals with the actual and is well-anchored to earth, enjoying the present	May not be in the present as may be anticipating what might happen; has 'head in the clouds'
Facts are important and should be used; may not look for possibilities	Ideas and possibilities are more interesting; may miss important facts
Likes to do things, and relaxes by doing things too	Likes to think things up
Usefulness is appealing	Creativity is appealing
Notices precise and detailed things; may lose sight of the whole picture	Tends to notice the whole rather than the details, and may be unobservant
May see iNtuitive types as somewhat giddy-minded, impractical and unrealistic	May see Sensing types as somewhat boring, and unable to grasp ideas
Needs to develop some iNtuition for balance	Needs to develop some Sensing qualities for balance.

American figures tell us that Sensing is present in 75 per cent of the general population, and iNtuition in 25 per cent. Further, we can expect equal numbers of male and female Ss and Ns in the general population. Since the Ss are much greater in number that the Ns, we can see that Ss are more at home in the world around them. Like Is, Ns are in the minority, and frequently feel out-of-step with what goes on in society.

Misunderstandings between people are caused by differences in all four pairs of preferences, but the S and N differences in the way we perceive things probably cause us the greatest frustration and disagreement. As Ss need to know about things through one of their five senses, this means they literally need to see, touch, feel, taste or smell something, otherwise it does not exist for them. For Ns things exist quite happily in their imaginations, they do not need to make things concrete. INtuitives can turn over ideas and concepts in their minds, linking one thing to another. When Ss and Ns communicate information to each other they may have difficulty in understanding what the other says.

Sensers may feel iNtuitives are careless and irresponsible about checking and noticing facts and details; Ns may feel Ss are unimaginative and unable to see or think ahead. If an S is taking directions from an N they may find they have not been given the detailed step-by-step information they need, the N saying something like: 'It's up the corridor, past that round thing, and somewhere on the left'. The S is likely to be more specific, saying: 'As you leave the lift on the second floor you turn right up the corridor. You pass the nurse's office which has a circular bay, and Dr Smith's office is the third door on the left'.

Another N, however, stands a good chance of understanding the N's directions. INtuitives can talk to one another without finishing sentences, yet other Ns can know and understand what they mean. This is an enigma to the S who likes to be given every specific detail.

Friends of mine are an S husband and an N wife. They live in a large house and often need to tell one another where something is. He, as an S, might say: 'It's on the left hand side of the right hand shelf in the DIY cupboard on the second floor'. She panics – too many instructions cause chaos in an N's mind – but in any case she needs it the other way round: 'It's on the second floor in the DIY cupboard, the right hand shelf and on the left'. The S has gone from the specific (the precise position of the object) to the general (the second floor), whereas the N goes from the general (the second floor) and then moves to the specific (the precise position of the object).

Sensers cope with practical living more easily than iNtuitives. They usually find it easier to do things around the house and to manage the mundane details of daily life. They generally cope with practical living more easily, without this draining their energy too much. INtuitives have more difficulty with this. Because we live in a concrete and practical world Ns have to learn how to cope with living in it. Some manage better than others, but many Ns use up a lot of energy doing this, needing more time to accomplish basic daily tasks, often leaving themselves exhausted and drained.

Sometimes Ns wonder why they are drained, as they feel they have not been doing much; often this is because they are using up a lot of energy in coping with practical details – the practicalities of keeping and organizing a home, travelling, driving, cooking, shopping, sewing, remembering where they have their keys and getting to the right place at the right time may all take their toll on an N. If they have to follow complex directions they may worry that they may not retain these in their minds. They are having to draw on their less developed S side for these. Of course Ss can get drained doing these things too, but they are less likely to do so as they are living out of their better developed side.

Sensers have a greater capacity for enjoying the physical pleasures of the world, as they are more fully present in the moment. INtuitives tend to be restless to move on to the next moment, often failing to enjoy the present.

Sensers' conversation often makes reference to facts from the past, but with no particular need to relate them to the future. For the N the past is past, and when Ns make reference to history it is usually with the idea of using the facts for the future.

We can see that both types of Perceiving are valuable, depending on what sort of information we are looking for. When we are making important decisions it may be helpful to check with an opposite Type before deciding – it is likely to bring to our attention information we may not think of. This way we have more balanced perception, giving us wider and more accurate data on which to make up our minds.

Sometimes people feel they ought to be balanced between the two, but this does not seem to be a good thing. When we are aware of either S or N dominating we know how we are functioning and can go ahead and use this in our life. If we are in no man's land – in the middle – we may not know where our strengths and preferences are, and subsequently do not know out of which function we are working.

If you feel you are in the middle there may be times when you experience difficulties in life. There are reasons why we may not have developed any of our natural preferences – and one reason is that we may have had one or more of these preferences suppressed in childhood. In adult life we may never have developed our true function. Yet it is never too late for any of us to take steps, even if they are small ones, towards becoming our true selves, and as we read on we will find a clearer picture emerges of this.

Thinking and Feeling

These, our Judging Functions, tell us how we make our decisions, and how we come to conclusions and judgements about things. In order to make our decisions we first need to take in information from our Perceiving functions, S or N, and we have read about the different ways we do this. When we have acquired our information in our S or N manner our decision is made on what we have absorbed. We cannot make decisions on information we have not taken in, and we need to understand that people not only make decisions differently (Thinking and Feeling) but they also make them on different information (S and N).

As with the different functions S and N, we have different ways of making decisions, and feel more comfortable making them with our preferred function.

We make our decisions with our preferred function of Thinking or Feeling. Our Thinking (T) function uses rational and logical thought, and is more firm minded, detached and impersonal. People with a preference for Thinking (T) can generally view a situation from outside, feeling less personally involved. Thinkers are less likely to show their feelings – although they have very strong feelings – and they can be objective. Good at analysing, they usually stand firm on their decisions, and are less likely to be swayed by human emotions.

Our Feeling (F) function places more importance on considering harmony in human relationships, being affected by people's needs and circumstances, personal feelings and loyalty. Feeling types identify with the emotions of others and their decisions are based on how these influence people for good or bad. When thinking something over a Feeling type considers: 'How does this affect people?'

The Thinking (T) type believes more in fairness and justice, and speaks out and gets incensed by unfairness and injustice. When decisions need to be talked through this is done methodically and coolly. Extenuating circumstances are not usually given much consideration by the T, who values standards and principles.

The Feeling (F) type makes decisions more personally and subjectively, and is persuaded by human needs and situations. Feelers are likely to show their feelings more and express sympathy. Unlike Ts, they feel personally involved in most decisions, and may go out of their way to please someone.

Here are some statements relating to each function.

Thinking function	Feeling function
Likely to make decisions ruled by head, choosing impersonally and objectively	Likely to make decisions with the heart, swayed more by personal and subjective values
Can see a point from a logical and rational angle	Sees human needs as being paramount
Good at analysing, and admires firm principles	Considers sympathy and harmony to be more important
Reacts emotionally as much as a Feeling type but less likely to show feelings, so many think person not feeling anything	Feelings show
Works for firm or company; able to stand outside situations and be reasonably unemotional	Works for a boss and the people in the company; feels involved in most situations and tries to preserve harmonious human relationships
Likely to take a firm stand on most issues	Likely to be persuaded by personal needs on most issues
May feel Feeling types are muddle-headed and illogical	May feel Thinking types are cold and inhuman
Can benefit from considering other people's feelings and looking at the human situations	Can benefit from seeing reason and logic. May be helpful to check with a Thinking type when making a decision

Thinkers (Ts) and Feelers (Fs) may find that they don't misunderstand one another so much as disagree with one another. Thinkers can feel that Fs are fuzzy-minded about their decisions, while Fs may feel Ts appear hard-hearted and cold.

Thinkers are likely to shrug their shoulders and say, 'Tough' when hearing about an unfortunate situation, while Fs are likely to give sympathetic looks and say, 'Poor thing'. Yet Ts have feelings just as much as Fs, they are just less likely to show them. Feelers' feelings are often quite apparent, showing quite clearly in their faces and bodies.

It seems that people have equal preferences for making T or F judgements, 50 per cent for both. But here there is the one and only difference between men and women: around 65 per cent of men prefer T, and only 35 per cent of women; whereas 65 per cent of women prefer

F, and only 35 per cent of men. This male/female difference gives us an expectation in our society that males should be governed more by their heads and females more by their hearts.

A typical scenario is the T male urging the F female to 'Try and be logical for once', while the F female might say to the T male: 'Try and share your feelings with me for once'. This is the more usual scenario as we have more T men and more F women. But when the situation is reversed, which happens less frequently, this may go against our cultural grain. In spite of the advent of the 'New Man', who is expected to show F behaviour, we are not always accepting of either him or the T woman. Society still expects them both to show their opposite characteristics as well as their natural ones.

Thinkers, whether male or female, are more able to face telling other people unpleasant things, and are likely to speak out truthfully even when this may not be tactful. They are less concerned with putting themselves across as likeable people.

Feelers on the other hand, try hard to avoid telling other people unpleasant things, and may fight shy of the truth in order to be tactful. Feelers want people to like them, and many of them look for opportunities where they can express themselves in an F manner, thereby receiving other people's warmth and approbation.

For example, the T is more capable of informing someone they are to be made redundant, and while they may not enjoy doing this they are less likely to be disturbed by it. The F is likely to find this task most disagreeable, and may try to get someone else to do this. If Fs are obliged to tell someone at work they are to be made redundant they may feel personally involved and share the misery of the other person's feelings.

Thinkers and Feelers can live and work together more easily when each type can explain their points of view to the other. Thinkers can see that Fs can understand and grasp a logical viewpoint, and Fs can see that Ts have deep feelings, even if they are not visible. If Ts are prepared to consider people's feelings and wishes, and Fs are prepared to consider the logical consequences of a decision, then there is a better chance of agreement between the two. Both can feel that their viewpoints are taken into account.

Judging and Perceiving

This pair of preferences tell us about another of our attitudes to living. They relate to whether we are more comfortable using our Perceiving function of Sensing or iNtuition, or our Judging function of Thinking or Feeling.

Do you like to spend more time taking in information and perceiving the world around you, or do you spend more time making decisions or judgements about the world? People who prefer the Judging attitude tend to be happier when life is planned and well organized. They usually make decisions easily, and like to carry out these decisions without changing them. When they wake up in the morning they prefer to know what they are going to do, and if the arrangements are changed they may get upset and flustered. Judgers like their lives to have a purpose, and find it hard to adjust to unexpected or changing situations.

People who prefer the Perceiving attitude are more easy-going, needing less of a framework to life, as they make their decisions as the need arises. Decisions are often delayed in order to collect more data or 'see what happens', and decisions may be left until the last moment – something that makes a Judger extremely anxious! When they wake in the morning Perceiving types are happy to feel the day can unfold, possibly bringing surprises. If the unexpected turns up or situations change Ps adapt well to these, going with the flow of life.

The two attitudes, Judging (J) and Perceiving (P), are opposing ways of living. The organized Judging type plans ahead, makes preparations and completes projects on time. Days are spent constructively and creatively, seldom wasted or idled away. Judgers often feel a sense of urgency, as they are always moving towards completing a project, whether this is getting a meal or writing a thesis. Incompleted tasks are always in the J's mind and s/he is not happy until the task is completed.

The less organized and more flexible Perceiving Type makes few definite plans, and these are subject to alteration and change. Preparations are not generally made, Ps preferring to do things as they go along. Less sense of urgency is felt, as Ps like to gather more information rather than feel they need to finish the project. This usually results in a number of projects on the go simultaneously, unlike Js who prefer to tackle one thing at a time. Perceivers are happy to experience life, and are less concerned with achievements.

Whereas Js feel unsettled when a project is incomplete Ps may feel unsettled after completing a project, feeling they have closed something and that it is final and unalterable.

About 55 per cent of the general (American) population are Judgers and 45 per cent Perceivers. Males and females are equally represented.

Judging Attitude	Perceiving Attitude
Prefers to get things settled	Prefers to have things open and fluid, to go with the flow of life
Makes deadlines and keeps to them; prefers to keep to arrangements once made	Deadlines are a reminder of what needs doing; may change arrangements
Feels better when decisions have been made, can then get on	May put off making a decision in order to collect more data; can feel uneasy when a final decision is made
Works hard and reliably; prepares for jobs and clears up afterwards; seldom relaxes unless work is done	Works hard too, but prefers to work when in the mood; not keen on preparation or clearing up. Happy to play or relax even if there is work to do
Plans and structures life and likes others to do the same; can be thrown if plans have to be changed	More flexible, and reluctant to be pinned down; good at adapting to whatever happens
Often has a sense of urgency, and likes to get on with things	Usually feels there is plenty of time; quite happy to wait and see
Feels Perceiving types can be indecisive, aimless and purposeless	Feels Judging types can be driven, task-oriented and inflexible
Can benefit from being open to further information and being more flexible	Can benefit by developing more structure and order

We can see how Judgers and Perceivers are attracted to each other, yet may drive each other up the wall! The J benefits from the P's playfulness and spontaneity – Js tend not to be spontaneous, being more organized people – and the Ps benefit from the J's ability to bring order and structure to life. Many relationships work this way, the P bringing fun and adaptability to the relationship and the J taking on the job of organizing things for both of them.

Anna (a J), finding that her husband was to be away on the following weekend, tried to bring structure to the weekend by organizing a visit to two of her friends. Both of them were Ps. Anna pressed for a

18

specific time with both of them, wanting to put this in her diary, but neither of the Ps were prepared to commit themselves in advance – one saying she 'wasn't sure' what she would be doing, and the other saying she would need to 'wait and see' until nearer the time. Anna got frustrated as both Ps spent considerable time on the phone going over all the possibilities for the weekend. Judgers tend to be quicker to come to decisions and arrangements, so Anna was most frustrated as she felt her friends had both been unfocused and indecisive, leaving her with indefinite plans – something that is unsettling for a J.

Perceivers who may be obliged to work in structured jobs that require clocking in and out at specific times, may find the evenings and weekends are their only chance to be more open-ended and flexible. When seen at work they may appear more J, but when seen at home they may be quite different, being more relaxed, easy-going and spontaneous.

As soon as Bryony (a J) got together with Alan (a P), her boyfriend, she was getting out her diary, making dates for the week ahead, the month ahead and even the following year! This was too much for Alan, whose job demanded that he be organized and work to time during the week, and at weekends he would make no plans until he got up, and often not even then. The more Bryony pressed him to fill his diary up the more Alan backed away from committing himself. In his spare time he liked to feel he had left his choices open. Having choices is important to Ps.

In the end Alan felt pressurized and Bryony felt thwarted. They agreed that neither was able to meet the other's strong J and strong P needs and they would be best apart. With an understanding of the other's attitude they have remained friends.

Judgers tend to shut off their willingness to receive more information once they have made a decision. This can sometimes be a mistake as it may prevent them from taking in some vital information. Perceivers, on the other hand, may continue to collect data without doing anything with it.

This chapter lets us know a number of things about ourselves and others:

Extraversion and **Introversion** tell us whether we have an outer or inner *attitude* to the world

Sensing and **iNtuition** tell us how we *perceive* the world around us. Perceiving is a way in which we *function*

Thinking and **Feeling** tell us how we come to *Judgement* about our perceptions. Judging is a way in which we function

Judging and **Perceiving** tell us whether we are more comfortable with our judging or perceiving function; these are attitudes to the world

When we know which *preference* is stronger in us we know our Type. If we are, for example, more Extraverted than Introverted, more Sensing than iNtuitive, more Thinking than Feeling and more Judging than Perceiving our Type is Extraverted-Sensing-Thinking-Judging (ESTJ). If you are Introverted, iNtuitive, Feeling and Perceiving your type is INFP.

The way this can be seen is illustrated below by Beryl Shedden.

Eating Cherry Cake

Extraverts will need to talk (possibly with mouth full if a P but not a J) about the cake and everything else, unless tired or they've come to the end of what interests them.

Introverts will eat in silence if INT or if they have come straight from discussion. If ISTs have come from being alone they may talk while eating, but not necessarily about what the Es are talking about.

Sensors will notice that it is *cherry* cake and savour the taste; the ESs will comment about this even if it is stating the obvious. SJs may eat the cake first and keep the cherries until last but they will be more likely to eat it 'properly' as it comes. SPs will eat the cherries first if they like them best.

INtuitives may not necessarily notice that it *is* cherry cake, but will certainly be wondering what sort of cake is planned for tomorrow, and will be picking up from the atmosphere whether everyone is enjoying what they are actually chewing!

Thinkers will be thinking about cherry cake. STs will probably be working out the recipe and considering what other recipes could equally well be used. NTs may be thinking about something else entirely, such as will we be getting indigestion from whatever we are eating or does it add to my weight problem. If any of the Es comments have penetrated to the INTs (remember the INTPs will be impervious) INTJs may consider for a while and probably say quite clearly: 'People

---

should not make so much fuss about what they are eating; there are far more important considerations in life'!

Feelers will be aware in themselves of either pleasure or distaste, according to which they will be either happy or concerned for everyone else whom they are convinced will be feeling the same. If anyone shows *outwardly* the opposite to what the Fs are feeling they will get very distressed indeed. If FJ they will try to identify and get rid of what is bringing this disharmony into the group, and if EFJ probably ask the waitress for a choice to be made available. The ESFJ might go so far as to ask the complainers: 'Who prefers cake and who prefers the cherries?' and offer to swop one for the other (whether or not it's their *own* preference) so that grumblers get what they want and peace is restored.

Judgers will want to demonstrate the normal and acceptable way to eat cherry cake.

Perceivers will *enjoy* their cake, scooping up crumbs with moistened fingers!

and A GOOD TIME WAS HAD BY ALL!!!

By now you are probably getting a picture of your type. We will now go on to look at the 16 different types created by these preferences.

4

Profiles of the Different Personality Types

In this chapter we consider the profiles of the 16 types. First, however, we can remind ourselves of the characteristics we expect to find in each type. These are sufficiently clear to enable us to recognize these in ourselves and in those around us. Here are the type characteristics, very briefly:

Extraverts are more outgoing, talk easily and like to work and play with others
Introverts are more reserved, talk less and need to have more time alone

Sensers live in the present, rely on facts and handle practical matters well; like things to be definite and measurable
INtuitives are more creative and look to the future; prefer imagining possibilities and work towards improving things

Thinkers make decisions using logic and impersonal analysis; use their heads rather than their hearts
Feelers more people-oriented and like to consider human needs; use their hearts rather than their heads

Judgers like to be organized, working to complete projects
Perceivers like to be flexible, open to change as more information is collected

From these brief descriptions we can draw a quick picture of each type. For example an ESTJ type is outgoing, relies on facts, is logical and organized. And an INFP type is reserved, creative, people-oriented and flexible. Each type has particular characteristics that are unique to it. As well as reading about your own type in the following type profile, do read the description of your opposite type, as this lets us know some of the things we may find difficult.

Another point is to notice what proportion of the general population belongs to each Type.[1] All ES types, for example, live and work with plenty of others who share their characteristics, whereas all IN types are less likely to come into contact with others like themselves, sometimes causing them to feel a sense of isolation.

Extraverted–iNtuitive–Feeling–Judging (ENFJ)

Outgoing   Creative   People-oriented   Organized

A warm and caring manner with people and an ability to suggest and organize things makes ENFJs popular leaders of groups. If an ENFJ believes in something, s/he can generate enthusiasm, and the flowing speech and persuasive approach help others to respond to her/his ideas. ENFJs are responsive to others and this makes them popular.

These qualities bring success in many careers, and ENFJs are likely to be drawn to work that involves personal contact with people. Radio, television and the media attract ENFJs, and they make marvellous salespersons, bringing a personal involvement to the transaction. If ENFJs take up teaching in any form, they are well liked by both staff and pupils. ENFJs make good therapists. ENFJs are drawn to religious and spiritual matters, and may take an active part in groups of this nature. They find the practical administration side of any job irksome, and small details demoralizing. For this reason jobs like accountancy, insurance and banking are not attractive.

An ENFJ's life is invariably full: ENFJs commit themselves to many people and many projects. They always fulfil these commitments, which means they are frequently in a rush. This may be because they have not allowed enough time for each of the projects. Everyone is invited into an ENFJ's home, and given food and a warm welcome. The telephone is always ringing, and the phone bill likely to be high!

Too much time alone does not appeal to ENFJs as they function best with people around them. Being alone for too long may depress an ENFJ, and s/he will quickly fill in time by arranging to meet people; ENFJs are most sociable. Conflict and disharmony at work or at home are upsetting, and ENFJs will do almost anything to avoid these. They seldom speak an unkind word about anyone.

With such outstanding abilities in human relationships ENFJs naturally attract people. While they enjoy having people around them this also means that people tend to offload their problems. A strong feeling function immediately identifies with others' problems, making them an ENFJ's own. This can lead to an ENFJ becoming emotionally exhausted as s/he takes on other people's worries. Although the ENFJ will then need time for restoration, a deep sense of commitment may not allow this.

All types may let themselves down by being unaware of the possible importance of other characteristics. ENFJs may need to check they do not rush into things, that they have the facts, that they look at situations from a logical point of view and that they take new information into account before making decisions.

Around 4 per cent of the general population are ENFJs, and as they tend to be spread across a variety of occupations they may not meet too many of their own type. There are more female ENFJs than male.

Introverted–iNtuitive–Feeling–Judging (INFJ)

Reserved   Creative   People-oriented   Organized

INFJs are people with very deep feelings; they show concern and care for those around them. They have a strong desire to contribute to the personal development of others, and can be an inspiration to people.

But many people may not benefit from an INFJ's best qualities, as s/he tends not to open up to others unless s/he knows them well and can trust them. People may feel the INFJ is a nice person, but a trifle cool. INFJs are not at all cool and are governed by intense feelings, but many of their deepest and most complex thoughts and emotions may be retained within and never shared with others. An understanding EN type may instinctively know of this rich inner life, and may help the INFJ to bring this out for the benefit of those around her/him.

People can always rely on an INFJ to produce work on time, be punctual at meetings and to keep his/her word. Projects and work are tackled in good time – INFJs do not like a last minute rush. They hate breaking their word, and go to great lengths not to do this. They are conscientious and persevering, and at times needing to complete things is at war with the need to reflect, imagine and dream.

On many an occasion an INFJ will have an uncanny sense of what is going to happen to people, and is usually right. It cannot be explained how or why INFJs have these premonitions, but many do have psychic abilities. An INFJ's mind is generally whirling around with likely possibilities, and s/he is highly sensitive to criticism and conflict, going out of his/her way to avoid these.

INFJs need work that makes use of their ability to bring out the best in others. Teaching or one of the other caring professions often suits well, and students know they will be supported and encouraged to fulfil their potential. INFJs are likely to have been successful students themselves, having a talent for academic work. Art and music may also interest them. Understanding people fascinates INFJs, and they may take up psychiatry or psychology. Religion and spirituality have a great attraction, and they may choose work in this field.

Many INFJs are writers: this is how they are able to communicate some of their deep inner thoughts and feelings to other people. They may not be able to express their inner thoughts verbally, but in writing have amazing fluency and powers of communication. Clearly not all INFJs write for a living – though many do – but most write for their own enjoyment or as part of their work or social life. Others go into the world of publishing.

INFJs may need to check that they do not spend too long considering matters, that they have the facts, look at situations from a logical viewpoint, and that they take new information into account before making decisions.

Only 1 per cent of people are INFJs and there are rather more females than males. An INFJ may not meet too many of her/his own kind, but will meet some as they all share clearly defined interests.

Extraverted–iNtuitive–Feeling–Perceiving (ENFP)

Outgoing   Creative   People-oriented   Flexible

ENFPs are likely to have a full and varied lifestyle, and it is usual for them to take up several careers in their lifetime. ENFPs bring warmth and enthusiasm to their work, and with their imaginative and ingenious minds turn their abilities to almost anything that attracts them. Others are encouraged by their cheerful and humane attitude and this makes them generally popular.

In any work, ENFPs need involvement with people; and they do not work well on their own for long. ENFPs love to initiate ideas for business and new projects, and talk in a convincing manner so that others are enthused to give support. Great pains are then taken to present projects both verbally or in writing, and numerous people are approached who could be involved. However, when a project starts to get off the ground and small practical details need attending to, ENFPs become restless and are less keen, and unless there is someone to see to these more S details the ENFP's excellent project may die the death. As such, ENFPs are better starters than finishers, and more organized types wonder why a brilliant start often comes to a dead end.

Although ENFPs will tackle concrete practical work on a temporary basis – and due to their adaptable nature and ability to improvise may be quite successful – they tend to be drawn to work with more human interaction. In sales and advertising they are certainly successful, and psychology and teaching are of interest. Acting also makes use of an ENFP's talents. In business ENFPs are encouraging to colleagues and staff, seldom playing the heavy boss.

As a partner ENFPs are fun, gentle and likeable. Male and female ENFPs can charm with no effort. A smile, personal glance and a kiss blown their way ensures the other person is caught! Living with an ENFP may work well for another P partner, but a strong J may find the ENFP unpredictable, as s/he may spend money impulsively on expensive luxuries.

Exhaustion can overtake the ENFP frequently as s/he sees the daily events of life as full of meaning and significance. The ENFP mind is constantly whirling around, fitting in each new piece of information, and may become overloaded and depressed. As they are on the go all the time, ENFPs' energy gets depleted, and they need affirmation from others in order to continue. They are generally most perceptive about people, but at times may move on to draw the wrong conclusions about these perceptions. ENFPs have masses of friends and colleagues, and their phone book is crammed with names. People know they can always contact an ENFP if they need to be put in touch with someone.

ENFPs may need to check that they do not rush into things, have the facts, look at situations from a logical viewpoint, and that they do not delay decisions too long or miss deadlines.

About 4 per cent of the general population are ENFPs. Since they move around so much they are likely to meet others of their type, but as long as they have a new project on hand and are surrounded by accepting people they are generally content.

Introverted–iNtuitive–Feeling–Perceiving (INFP)

Reserved   Creative   People-oriented   Flexible

INFPs are unusual people, being highly sensitive and intuitive. They often contribute in a generous and extensive manner to their chosen interests. Vast amounts of knowledge, perceptions and possibilities are within them, and these are often communicated in teaching or writing. In day-to-day interaction some people may see INFPs as reserved and unsociable, so they may be misjudged.

INFPs believe very strongly in contributing to the benefit of people in the world around them, and may commit themselves loyally to a variety of projects, finding they are continually hard pressed to complete these. They may find they are running late throughout the day as they may not be well-organized – often due to an inability to assess the time needed for each task. Easy-going people may get used to INFPs being late, but those who are well-organized themselves dislike this.

The INFP's strong ideals sometimes conflict with the realities of daily life. If they choose a partner who is down-to-earth and realistic the partner is likely to see to all the small practical details of life. A partner who is similar to the INFP may mean that the two of them pay little attention to the practicalities of this world and spend their time exchanging ideas and concepts without putting them into action.

As a child the INFP naturally took in information and knowledge, usually making a good student. Research work suits INFPs as they are patient in collecting details, and enjoy anything connected with the development of people. Counselling, psychiatry and psychology is of interest, and they are likely to be drawn to religious and spiritual spheres. Musical people are often INFPs, as are artists. INFPs can be gifted at languages, and this includes the language of the computer. If they turn to the commercial world they succeed best if they have responsibility for the welfare of staff, for example in personnel.

The INFP's belief in goodness and light is touched with a strand of melancholy. They are acutely aware of the darker side of life, and this may drag them into episodes of deep depression when others can barely reach them. It takes a wise and profound partner to understand the INFP.

Life is an ongoing quest for meaning for the INFP, and they may have a sense of isolation at times as they may not meet many of their own type. Their sense of having a unique contribution to use in the world becomes desperately frustrated if they are unable to find an outlet for this.

INFPs may need to check that they do not spend too long considering matters, that they have the facts, look at situations from a logical viewpoint, and that they do not delay decisions too long or miss deadlines.

About 1–2 per cent of the general population are INFPs, with more females than males. This may mean they feel separated from and unlike the rest of the population.

Extraverted–iNtuitive–Thinking–Judging (ENTJ)

Outgoing Creative Logical Organized

People of this type are frank and outspoken, and communicate in a direct and straightforward manner. Other people are seldom left in any doubt as to what is meant. This manner may come across as somewhat aggressive to types of a milder disposition, but ENTJs have a need to explain and clarify things clearly to other people. ENTJs' organizational powers are formidable, especially concerning the use of time and cost-effective ways of using people. This is why they are often appointed to a managerial position.

Much of the ENTJ lives through work, and s/he is unstinting in what

27

s/he does, expecting others to be the same. After people have let an ENTJ down more than once, they are monitored and their work checked.

Talkative, articulate and usually confident, ENTJs are often seen as down-to-earth and practical. People are surprised to find that above all they have a drive to create, to bring into force something new, to do something that has not been done before. Routine administration and small details are of little interest to ENTJs, but they will push themselves to do these if it leads to the end-product they are wanting.

Since ENTJs may climb the managerial ladder quickly, they can find themselves in charge of other people – possibly groups of people. As a general rule, leadership comes naturally to ENTJs, and they are happy to give directives to others, and do any public speaking. Others, however, may see the ENTJ as bossy.

When asked their opinion ENTJs invariably bring logic to their reply. If an answer is not logical it carries no weight with them. People who express themselves emotionally without logic get little attention from ENTJs; but if something can be seen to be logical as well as emotional they can be understanding and empathetic.

Very independent by nature, ENTJs plan well ahead and like to be in control of what they do and when they do it. Quiet, sensitive and less organized types may find them overpowering and forceful, and ENTJs may need to approach people like these more gently.

ENTJ males usually find it easier to be accepted in our society than ENTJ females. At home, both males and females expect all family members to pull their weight and to be organized. If their domestic or day-to-day family life makes excessive demands on them this may be irksome, as they need outlets for more creative projects.

ENTJs may need to check that they do not rush into things, that they have the facts, consider other people's feelings, and that they take new information into account before making decisions.

They may not come into contact with a large number of their own type – which is around 4 per cent of the general population – as all are busy putting plans into action! They can expect to meet more males than females.

Introverted–iNtuitive–Thinking–Judging (INTJ)

Reserved   Creative   Logical   Organized

The INTJs forward thinking and creative mind is always engaged in working out some new project. Even if things appear to be working well, the INTJ is unlikely to be content, and can invariably see a way to improve things. Wherever possible INTJs see that their plans are put into action.

At work, INTJs are likely to be seen as original people who can look to the future and plan for it. And their drive to bring this change and improvement at all levels is backed up by good organizational powers in seeing projects through.

Trivial and mundane family matters are of no interest to INTJs, and on social occasions they may have little to say. This can be seen by others as impolite and stand-offish, but INTJs are just not interested in the domestic details of daily life. On social occasions INTJs may offer a remark, possibly a genuine suggestion to improve life, and others may find this idea outrageous and bizarre; this may be because they cannot follow what is in the INTJ's original mind.

Many of the INTJs thoughts may not be expressed to others as they are reserved persons, and their creative thinking is an internal process. Rational thought is important to INTJs and everything they work on needs to be based on logic – even fun and play. When something appears logical and they can see in their minds it can be put into action, they will then work extremely hard to make it happen.

Most independent people, INTJs quietly go their own way, creating systems based on classifying and deducing and being able to demonstrate their worth. Although they prefer to work on their own ideas, they also have the ability to make sense of the ideas of others. They are then capable of putting forward these ideas in a comprehensible manner.

At work, INTJs are usually valued since there are few people of their type, and they can work in a number of spheres, provided they are responsible for forward planning. INTJs can be critical and stubborn. They are good with computers and can create new systems; they enjoy planning the best way of using people rather than products.

If a partner is an N type the INTJ is likely to be able to share many ideas and thoughts, but a partner of a more practical type may not be able to understand these; s/he will, however, let the INTJ know if the ideas will work out in practical terms.

INTJs may need to check that they do not spend too long considering matters, that they have the facts, consider people's feelings, and that they take new information into account before making decisions.

Only 1 per cent of the general population are the INTJ type, so many may feel a bit of a loner. There are more male than female INTJs.

Extraverted–iNtuitive–Thinking–Perceiving (ENTP)

Outgoing   Creative   Logical   Flexible

ENTPs are involved in numerous activities, and usually have an enormous variety of interests and projects on the go. Their tremendous capacity for generating ideas extends to most things that come their way. As they go about, ideas come to them from moment to moment, and their minds are a mass of ideas constantly whirling around. ENTPs move around from project to project all the time, and as they do, their ideas change as new information comes up.

Other people, especially the more J types, may find this a bit disconcerting at times; if they have started to follow a path or direction in a particular way, and the ENTP then comes back and says s/he now thinks something different, the person may be confused. ENTPs are resourceful and their thoughts move so quickly that few people are able to keep up with them.

ENTPs are good at presenting their ideas in such a way that others are keen to take them up. But they may not have thought through whether their ideas work out in practical terms, as they prefer to leave this to other people. Once their ideas have started to get off the ground – which usually requires attending to small practical details – ENTPs tend to lose interest and move on to the next thing. Hopefully someone else will continue to carry through their first idea or it will fall by the wayside. The importance of seeing to small practical details in a systematic manner may go unnoticed by ENTPs, and many a good idea of theirs has remained dormant because of this. But they are brilliant at getting things off the ground.

If they are tied to work or a home life that is based on routine and repetitive humdrum jobs ENTPs are desperately frustrated, and may get depressed without understanding why. ENTPs require considerable challenge and variety to their lives, needing a number of different projects to give their attention to. Other types may not understand this and may see ENTPs as uncommitted.

At work and on social occasions ENTPs are an entertaining and fascinating talker, being gregarious and generally good humoured. With their logical minds, they can argue for the merits of virtually anything they set their minds on – no one stands a chance when they are around!

ENTPs are unlikely to be a model of tidiness but they provide a lively environment for other family members. Not being interested in domestic trivia, ENTPs are good at organizing others to get this done. And they are full of ideas for ways of stretching children's minds, which means life is never dull. Designing new gadgets is another ENTP talent.

ENTPs may need to check that they do not rush into things, that they have the facts, consider people's feelings and that they do not delay decisions too long or miss deadlines.

Around 4 per cent of the general population are ENTP. ENTPs are likely to meet others of their type as they have an immense collection of friends and acquaintances. There are more male ENTPs than female.

Introverted–iNtuitive–Thinking–Perceiving (INTP)

Reserved   Creative   Logical   Flexible

INTPs bring logical and rational thought to all their opinions, and are usually considered to have intellectual superiority. This is because their minds quickly collect important data relating to the subject in hand, discarding anything irrelevant. INTPs are frequently one step ahead of others who may not be able to follow their complex reasoning.

As INTPs receive new information and ideas their minds immediately adapt to these, and present thoughts and decisions change around to fit in. This is done happily – indeed INTPs enjoy doing this, feeling that everything in life continues to alter and expand. Problems are generally seen as situations that emerge and develop, not as set and rigid circumstances needing a specific response.

However, putting ideas into action is another story, as these notions may be somewhat far-fetched or impractical. INTPs are unlikely to put ideas into practice as their minds race ahead to the next thing that catches their attention. Others who have the ability to follow through on INTP ideas may be credited with the original idea.

Since INTPs live largely in the world of abstract thought and ideas, they may be seen as withdrawn, detached and eccentric. Often they are avid readers devouring book after book, and people may wonder if they are ever in the real world! INTPs let the 'real' world get on with its business; they have their own theoretical world.

A job that makes use of INTP abilities may be hard to find, and INTPs are often happiest in research, where they can continually add new information to their findings. Work that demands a set routine and too much practical detail is not for INTPs, and they are less likely to be successful with this. Any work they undertake needs to allow INTPs to research all avenues around the subject, not necessarily coming up with an instant answer. In our society male INTPs are given greater acceptance than females – who may be looked upon as somewhat unfeminine nonconformists.

As a family member the INTP tends to keep away from too much domestic and social life – unlike the opposite type, ESFJ. But INTPs are generally easy-going and happy to let family life go on around them, not being bothered by untidiness or the lack of regular meals. Looking after the home on a regular basis does not appeal, and INTPs do not see the need for this. If they have children, INTPs like them to develop their minds, not just their skills, and INTPs may make special opportunities for this.

INTPs may need to check that they don't spend too long considering matters, that they have the facts, consider people's feelings, and that they do not delay decisions too long or miss deadlines.

With around 1 per cent of the general population being INTPs contact with many others of the same type is unlikely – especially as they are inclined to a rather solitary lifestyle.

Extraverted–Sensing–Thinking–Judging (ESTJ)

Outgoing   Literal   Logical   Organized

ESTJs are down-to-earth, well-rooted and practical people. They are aware of what is going on in the world around them as they are usually in the middle of this. Straightforward and direct, people know where they are with ESTJs, and at work they expect people to be reliable and productive. ESTJs have high standards and expect other people to have these too.

Ideas and theories are only considered useful to ESTJs if they can see how they work out in practice. If they feel something will result in a useful end-product they are likely to support it, otherwise the idea is dismissed as unworkable.

ESTJs' outgoing nature means that they are usually in-touch and up-to-date with current, business and local news, and they often learn about these by talking to others. People find ESTJs a mine of information as they can always produce a mass of relevant facts about the world. Because of this, they stand out in a crowd, speaking volubly and knowledgeably about things.

ESTJs are systematic and decisive, and their drive to see projects through makes them successful in many commercial areas. They do well in business and finance, often acquiring money and investing it wisely. In management, they are likely to rise to a high position as they get through a lot of work in the time available and can supervise others to do the same – being good and fairly tough administrators. As organizers ESTJs are outstanding and always reliable; people know they will carry a project through to the end.

Life is comparatively clear and simple for ESTJs, and they are candid and frank. Esoteric fields and conceptual theories may make them feel uneasy and be perplexing, and other types, of a more complex and idealistic nature, may find ESTJs a bit blunt. People's feelings take second place to getting a job done, whether this is at home or at work. On committees ESTJs may take the chair – others accepting their leadership of the group. Irresponsible people get short shrift from ESTJs as they have little patience with them.

At home, ESTJs make for outspoken but stable partners and parents. Others in the family know what to expect from them. ESTJs like a well-ordered and maintained home, and like people in it to be the same. ESTJs are likely to get involved in a number of projects in their community, where they enjoy taking an active role.

ESTJs may need to check that they don't rush into things, that they look ahead to future possibilities, consider people's feelings, and that they take new information into account before making decisions.

About 14 per cent of the general population are ESTJs. ESTJs meet plenty of people of their own kind – which is one reason why they feel at home in the material world.

Introverted–Sensing–Thinking–Judging (ISTJ)

Reserved Literal Logical Organized

ISTJs are found in professions like banking, insurance, law and accountancy. Such professions require people who can work on their own, deal with practical details in a logical manner and work to a routine. ISTJs are dominant in most branches of the Forces, and are suited to the strict and regimented life. They are also the backbone of many traditional institutions, going quietly about their business, conscious of their duty, and always fulfilling this. They make good and thorough supervisors.

Others may not recognize or value what ISTJs do, as they may come across as somewhat straight-laced and dull. ISTJs are willing to spend hours seeing to small practical details which other types may have little patience with. Conscientious and meticulous, ISTJs check and monitor facts with accuracy and concentration. Much of ISTJs' lives are taken up this way, especially if they feel responsible for the work. To be seen as responsible is a high priority with ISTJs.

ISTJs live their lives with inward concentration, and their minds are habitually centred on the steps necessary to achieve the completion of the task in hand. If they are convinced of the rightness of what they are doing nothing distracts them from this, and they speak out quite forcibly if necessary. People sometimes find ISTJs somewhat un-approachable as they may not have an easy-going manner. But people soon get to know they can depend on ISTJs to be utterly reliable. ISTJs get their information about the world around them by reading the newspapers thoroughly and regularly, and by listening to radio and TV.

At social gatherings ISTJs will not be described as the life-and-soul of the party – this is more likely to be said of their opposite type, ENFP. Ideas, fun and possibilities do not play a large part in ISTJ lives. But if ISTJs are asked the details of things which relate to their work or hobbies, they will produce a mass of accurate facts from way back right up to the present day. Some of the other types may not see the relevance of collecting facts about all sorts of apparently unrelated things, but ISTJs collect these by hearing or reading about them and they then store them up in their minds.

At work ISTJs are likely to arrive and leave at regular hours. Routine is an important framework for ISTJ lives.

Leisure may be spent belonging to traditional clubs or groups; these may range from Scouts or Guides to Rotary, Inner Wheel, Citizens Advice Bureaux, the Church, many community interests and sport. Esoteric groups are less likely to be of interest.

Female ISTJs tend to find fulfilment in the traditional role of wife and mother, and may feel lost in mid-life when children leave home, experiencing a sense of uselessness. Females are less likely than some of the other types to go out into the world and 'make their mark', and if they go out to work they experience some guilt about leaving their home responsibilities. All ISTJs are stable members of the family and everyone can rely on them.

ISTJs may need to check that they do not spend too long considering matters, that they look ahead to future possibilities, consider people's feelings, and that they take new information into account before making decisions.

At least 6 per cent of the general population are ISTJs, and as they tend to congregate with their own kind (and the ESTJs) they are unlikely to feel isolated. There are more male than female ISTJs.

Extraverted–Sensing–Feeling–Judging (ESFJ)

Outgoing   Literal   People-oriented   Organized

ESFJs are warm, outgoing, down-to-earth and well-organized, a type that most people are drawn to. They have a way of relating to people that makes them feel they are being cared for – whether it is taking their coat as they come into the home, cooking them a nourishing meal or asking after their welfare and seeing to their practical needs. Females find much fulfilment in their role in the home, often trying to prolong it by keeping the family at home and urging their return at weekends. Males are seen as caring parents in the same way.

ESFJs are very sociable and are usually great talkers, with plenty to say about the endless details of family life, or office details that involve the lives of the staff. For female ESFJs who are not able to have children there is usually much sorrow and disappointment.

Most people like ESFJs and speak warmly about them. ESFJs may go on with further education but their real forte is in giving a practical service to others. They tend to choose a business which provides for this. They may go into one of the service-to-people careers – nursing, teaching, reception work – anything that provides practical help for people. As a sales person they are outstanding, bringing a personal commitment and involvement to what they are selling.

ESFJs are likely to be involved on local committees, where they are recognized as co-operative and active members. Whether they are at home or at work, ESFJs extend themselves in looking after other people, and they may be undervalued by others taking them for granted. Because ESFJs are always good tempered, loyal and caring, people can forget to appreciate them. ESFJs need appreciation, and when given this they continue to give care and support to everyone. This is what life is about for ESFJs, and they have little interest in complex theories – the abiding concern of the INTPs, their opposite type. ESFJ females may feel abstractions are the province of men.

As a family member ESFJs remind other members of appointments and schedules, often accompanying them so they can arrive on time. Family life is filled with the busyness of home and family doings. These activities are then related to friends and colleagues with gusto, giving the details of each event. Often people will describe the ESFJ family as 'a marvellous united family' which may be due to the way the ESFJ gathers and looks after the family members.

Alternative lifestyles are not popular with ESFJs; they tend to feel these to be threatening to the status quo. Family members who act out of court are not popular either.

ESFJs may need to check that they do not rush into things, that they look ahead to future possibilities, look at situations from a logical viewpoint, and that they take new information into account before making decisions.

There are plenty of ESFJs in the general population, as many as 18 per cent, so they meet many people with whom they have much in common. There are more ESFJ females than males.

Introverted–Sensing–Feeling–Judging (ISFJ)

Reserved   Literal   People-oriented   Organized

Quiet, serious, painstaking, and hard-working describes the ISFJ. ISFJs seldom blow their own trumpet, and are rarely appreciated for what they do – often because others are quite unaware of their contributions. ISFJs frequently help behind the scenes and are seldom seen in the limelight.

ISFJs may work for years with the same organization, calmly and patiently carrying out a task which many other types might feel is boring. But ISFJs like their work to have a service-to-people aspect, feeling they are doing something useful to help others. If they are in jobs like accountancy, banking, and insurance ISFJs enjoy having personal contact with people. Female ISFJs are attracted to nursing, secretarial, reception work, catering and administrative work in medicine. They do these jobs with care and accuracy.

ISFJs do not need to be up-front, but their contribution needs to be recognized and appreciated. Leadership, fame and renown are not things they seek, and if they come their way ISFJs may not feel comfortable with them, finding it difficult to assume the position of boss. This can happen if they get promotion at work: whereas they were happy in the subordinate position, they may be less successful in a managerial position, and giving orders may be difficult for them. Others may be perplexed by this, as once they are promoted they expect ISFJs to give orders, and this may cause role confusion.

As a child the ISFJ was serious and obedient, the perfect child! As a parent, ISFJs are traditional, caring for and teaching their children the practical needs and steps of life. People soon get to know they can absolutely depend on ISFJs, and they may be taken for granted, given jobs that others would refuse, but ISFJs tend to take on a heavier load than they should do, always feeling it is their duty. Often extra efforts go unappreciated.

ISFJs are unlikely to do anything dramatic that catches the public eye. Their life carries on quietly. Because they are reserved they don't shout about what they do, and they can be gullible. Qualities like ingenuity, quick wittedness and whirlwind adaptability are not seen in them; these are the forte of the ISFJ's opposite type, ENTP. ISFJs are loyal and dependable, but not exciting, as a partner. Suggestions for spur-of-the-moment outings are not likely to come from ISFJs. If their partner is changeable and unpredictable the ISFJ is happy to provide the stable and practical base for them.

When children leave home the female ISFJ, if she is not employed, may feel she loses her identity, as much of her role may be bound up with the care of husband and children. As this role diminishes when children leave home a sense of uselessness may prevail. And if the marriage breaks up both male and female ISFJs feel the loss acutely, which is added to by their loss of role as husband or wife.

ISFJs are capable of doing a lot of practical work in a short time, and provided someone does not interrupt them and persuade them to do something else, they are a good time manager.

ISFJs may need to check that they do not spend too long considering matters, that they look ahead to future possibilities, look at situations from a logical viewpoint and that they take new information into account before making decisions.

At least 6 per cent of the general population are ISFJs, and they are likely to come across other ISFJs, together with plenty of ESFJs. There are more female ISFJs than male.

Extraverted–Sensing–Thinking–Perceiving (ESTP)

Outgoing   Literal   Logical   Flexible

People notice ESTPs, as they can be the focus of any gathering, always having something unusual to say. They can tell dramatic and interesting stories that have happened to them or other people, and they see to it that their lives have excitement and variety. Routine and the domesticity of daily life bore ESTPs quickly, and they frequently manage to escape this. This may be easier for males as they can create change through their work and through travel, which they love. ESTPs need to be active.

If their work includes too much repetition, ESTPs feel frustrated, and need to use their leisure time to do things on the spur of the moment. And if their work is not the 'hands on' variety then they like to do practical and active things in their spare time. ESTPs are good with their hands: they may paint realistically, do woodwork and sculpture, and enjoy DIY in the home when they feel like it. ESTPs can be musical, and if they play an instrument they enjoy using this in a variety of musical groups. ESTPs may enjoy sport.

Philosophy and psychology are not their scene. Ideas and theories, being things ESTPs are unable to get their hands on, are not too appealing to them. They are more concerned with the concrete and actual world around them. In fact, the concrete and actual of the present moment are what attracts ESTPs. They live for the moment, and as the moment changes so does their reaction to it. Some of the other types may feel they are changeable, possibly unreliable, but this is due to their sensitivity to small changes in life.

ESTPs are unlikely to be seen at groups for self-development, as delving into the unconscious is not of interest; they may be wary of more esoteric interests that 'tune into the vibes', perhaps not being aware of what 'the vibes' are!

Talkative on social occasions, ESTPs look for action rather than a heart to heart talk. Very grounded in present day realities, ESTPs base their decisions on facts; they make these decisions easily, logically and coolly, after having considered a variety of possibilities. If they are considering a project, they may follow up all the possibilities – not being upset if most of them come to nothing. For that reason ESTPs are always on the go, energetically chasing after something, often travelling somewhere, not staying in one place for too long. Male ESTPs, even in today's world, find it easier to have this lifestyle than their female counterparts. The female ESTP, who is left at home to be traditional wife and mother, will be frustrated from lack of excitement and variety, and needs to find some outlets for this.

Sensitive types may have difficulty in relating to ESTPs closely, as intimate ongoing relationships can drain and even embarrass them. The more they are pressed into this type of relationship the more they withdraw, both physically and emotionally. But for day-to-day casual friendships ESTPs are fun, companionable, easy-going and amiable. As a partner they can be exciting and unpredictable, but they bring a strong sense of realism to the relationship. The details of day-to-day family life do not attract ESTPs, and their urge to be off doing something new may mean they ignore these.

ESTPs are likely to be involved with a variety of work during their lives, bringing their talents to many things. Often they make their friends through their work. ESTPs enjoy work that is entrepreneurial, and they are sharp negotiators. They sail close to the wind and get restless for a bit of excitement. Machines, mechanical things and anything to do with transport – ships, planes and vehicles – attract ESTPs because they need operating and they move. When a business is in trouble ESTPs are just the people to turn losses into profit. But once the business is going well ESTPs lose interest in it. This is why they may initiate an excellent business, but in the end it may fail through lack of attention in maintaining it.

ESTPs may need to check that they do not rush into things, that they look ahead to future possibilities, consider people's feelings, and that they do not delay decisions too long or miss deadlines.

Like other ES types there are plenty of ESTPs – perhaps around 12 per cent – and they do not lack for company. There are more ESTP males than females.

Introverted–Sensing–Thinking–Perceiving (ISTP)

Reserved   Literal   Logical   Flexible

ISTPs may not say a lot, as they prefer action to words, but they have a good grasp of the concrete realities of this world. ISTPs are observant and notice small practical details – an asset in the business world. When opportunities arise ISTPs are aware of them, and usually know when to move in and act – seldom wasting energy on unnecessary action. As they tend not to go in for small talk or gossip, people are often unaware of how sharp and astute ISTPs are.

Practical abilities in ISTPs extend to an understanding and handling of mechanical things like machines and tools, vehicles and anything to do with transport. ISTPs have only to look at a machine or vehicle and get their hands on it to understand the way it works, and they often find work using these abilities. Taking a machine or vehicle apart, seeing how it works, repairing it and using it makes use of the ISTP's need for 'hands on' work. Any work that involves using their hands, or using machines and tools, suits ISTPs. Piloting a plane or driving a vehicle can bring satisfaction. But as a child parents and teachers may have despaired as the ISTP probably showed little interest in the more academic side of learning.

These qualities of being realistic and well-grounded give ISTPs a confidence and security with day to day practical living, something that other types may envy.

If their work provides ISTPs with excitement and variety, they are happy – working long hours, perhaps in discomfort, but with great endurance and skill. But if they are tied to a more mundane, formal or conventional job ISTPs get bored very quickly, and may try to create a drama or crisis to stir things up. Work needs to provide ISTPs with the challenge of using their skills of practical accuracy and precision in a changing environment. Fluctuations in business and commerce never upset ISTPs – they adapt to them easily, making use of their eagle eyes and quick wits.

The quiet life is not for them, and a traditional, repetitive job needs to be compensated for by spontaneous action at home. Spontaneity, impulsiveness and freedom to act are important to ISTPs – things that may puzzle a partner of a different type.

Although ISTPs may make commitments to a partner or at work, they are likely to keep these commitments to the minimum, as their greatest need is to be free. As they are highly tuned to small changes that happen from moment to moment, ISTPs prefer to be unhampered – they can then decide what to do as they go along.

The needs of male ISTPs are still given greater acceptance in society than those of female ISTPs. But female ISTPs are becoming more accepted now, which allows them to take up painting and decorating, work in the building trade, the transport industry, and to go into the Forces.

ISTPs may need to check that they do not spend too long considering matters, that they look ahead to future possibilities, consider people's feelings, and that they do not delay decisions too long or miss deadlines.

ISTPs, who comprise 6 per cent of the general population, are nevertheless scattered about, particularly at work. They are more likely to find similar types in their interests outside work.

Extraverted–Sensing–Feeling–Perceiving (ESFP)

Outgoing   Literal   People-oriented   Flexible

ESFPs are generally popular and people enjoy being in their company. Friendly to everyone, even to strangers, ESFPs are persuasive and talkative. Whether at home or at work they are likely to have many projects on at the same time, moving easily from one to another.

Theory and analysis hold little attraction for ESFPs, as they prefer to be in the thick of things, where the action is, rather than thinking about it. They are capable of attending to a number of practical tasks simultaneously as they have the gift of turning their concentration from one task to another as it is needed.

At home, ESFPs may have several projects started, but not finished. DIY interests ESFPs but may be left half-done if something else is more attractive. Meanwhile, the unfinished projects may not worry ESFPs as they are content to feel that they are in the process of being done; they may, however, worry a J partner who needs to see things completed.

People are welcomed into an ESFP's home – even if it is in a mess, and ESFPs provide a sociable and entertaining atmosphere, producing good food and talking away about a range of different activities. Often ESFPs can be dressed in flamboyant and trendy clothes, and they can make a fashion statement by knowing what clothes to mix and match together. ESFPs hate to miss anything that is going on and will try and pack several things into a short space of time. Since they are adaptable and thrive on one activity after another this may leave their partner or children gasping for a bit of peaceful home life.

A variety of sports may appeal to ESFPs and they make good coaches, being sensitive to the immediate and changing needs of their pupils. Teaching athletics and sport to classes, too, is a strength of ESFPs: they are likely to provide variety from week to week in order to keep their pupils' interest – and because of this, people enjoy coming to any group they are running.

By nature ESFPs are kind. Some ESFPs are comical and entertaining and may turn this into their profession. If their job requires travelling around they enjoy this and are happy to talk and chat to people they may never see again. Usually smiling or laughing, ESFPs can cheer people up. This can be useful in careers like nursing, as although ESFPs tend to find sadness and sorrow difficult to face, they are at their best in crisis work.

Routine and regulations pin ESFPs down too much as they like to react to the activities of the moment. ESFPs like to be doing something, not thinking about it. They enjoy public relations and make good salespersons – especially if they are selling a practical gadget or service. In business ESFPs excel in selling, knowing just the right thing to say at the right moment. Working in the theatre also appeals, as ESFPs love the excitement and drama.

ESFPs may need to check that they do not rush into things, that they look ahead to future possibilities, look at situations from a logical viewpoint, and that they do not delay decisions too long or miss deadlines.

ESFPs are found in a variety of professions, and as there are around 12 per cent of people of this type, they should meet others with reasonable frequency. There are more female ESFPs than male.

Introverted–Sensing–Feeling–Perceiving (ISFP)

Reserved   Literal   People-oriented   Flexible

ISFPs are often misunderstood as they are quiet, gentle and modest, seldom speaking out forcibly. They are most observant, noticing details from moment to moment, yet may not remark on them. They live right in the present moment, and when they are enjoying something it is hard to get them to move on to the next thing. Others may see ISFPs as people without direction in life, but in fact they are very much in touch with themselves and the world around them.

A natural with children and animals, ISFPs are strongly attuned to nature and the earth. 'Live and let live' is their motto, and they rarely seek to change people, believing that people and nature should live in harmony. This ability to feel at one with nature may lead to a desire to work out-of-doors, possibly with animals, farming or conservation.

ISFPs are often artistically gifted, possibly with dance, painting or music. And this is the way they express themselves to other people, rather than by talking to them. Long hours spent rehearsing or practising are not exhausting as this is 'doing' rather than preparing or planning. If this is done freely and impulsively their energy levels last beyond someone who forces themselves to work.

Graceful and co-operative, unusually kind and sympathetic, ISFPs are acutely aware of people's immediate needs, and are happy to provide for these. Sometimes they get so involved in the details of the present that they give little thought to the future. At work they react to the requirements of the moment, and in their homes guests are looked after with sensitivity. ISFPs care for people by seeing to their needs and providing them with carefully prepared meals. Children are given unfailing practical care, and they seem to know just when this is needed.

ISFPs need work that provides a service to people, but are not so keen on work that brings them up-front and into the limelight. Much of what ISFPs do may be behind the scenes, and it may go unnoticed and unthanked. Males are often told they are not forceful enough. Nursing or social work can provide what ISFPs need, as can the artistic realm and the outdoor world. ISFPs can be successful in clerical and practical hands-on work if they are given some day-to-day variety.

ISFPs may lag behind in class in school and some may find little attraction in academic subjects, not wishing to go on with further education. At school ISFP talents may not be spotted or appreciated, and people may be amazed in later life at their achievements.

ISFPs may need to check that they do not spend too long considering matters, that they look ahead to future possibilities, look at situations from a logical viewpoint, and that they do not delay decisions too long or miss deadlines.

In their chosen work and interests ISFPs may not meet many others of their type; there are around 6 per cent ISFPs in the general population, with more females than males.

From these profiles we can begin to develop some accuracy in predicting type, and in being realistic about what we expect from ourselves and everyone else. We become aware of the more positive aspects of each type, and this helps us to appreciate our own best qualities and those of other people. It also helps us to direct ourselves towards the best development for our type.

PROFILES OF THE DIFFERENT PERSONALITY TYPES

Now we have begun to understand something about the 16 types we can read on to see how our behaviour is governed by our *temperament*.

[1] The percentages given in the profiles are based on figures from the US but we can expect these to be similar in the UK.

5

Temperament:
Patterns to Our Behaviour

As we become aware of our own type we begin to notice different characteristics in those around us. We might, perhaps, become aware of a friend as being an I rather than an E; we might possibly also notice that he or she is a J rather than a P, but we do not necessarily become aware of all their preferences. It is easy to become confused about someone's type as there are many factors that affect the way in which we come across to others. We read more about how the different types behave in later chapters.

When we start learning about type most of us find that 16 variations are too many to contain in our minds. Fortunately, we now have a helpful method that gives us a shortcut to understanding the 16 types.

This method was discovered by an American, Professor David Keirsey, who has been researching differences in type for over 35 years. He tells us that as well as the different preferences that make up our type all of us have an *overall pattern* to our behaviour. This he calls our *temperament*.

Once we become aware of the four temperaments – our own and the three others – we find it easier to understand the 16 types. Since each temperament includes four types, we find that we have three other types in our temperament group. It can be encouraging for us to discover – especially if we are one of the less frequent types – that there are plenty of other people with whom we share thoughts, attitudes and behaviour, and this can give us a better base from which to work and live together.

This chapter lets us know how we can find our temperament, and some of the basic differences and driving forces of the four temperaments.

Finding our temperament

Once we have discovered our type it is a simple process to find our temperament. We do this by first taking our S or N function, whichever is our preference. If our preference is for N, for example, we link this to our T or F preference, giving us our temperament of NF or NT. If our preference is for S, we link this to our J or P preference, giving us our temperament of SJ or SP. We can see in the Table below which of the 16 types belong to each temperament.

NF	NT	SJ	SP
ENFJ	ENTJ	ESTJ	ESTP
INFJ	INTJ	ISTJ	ISTP
ENFP	ENTP	ESFJ	ESFP
INFP	INTP	ISFJ	ISFP

David Keirsey says: 'One's temperament is that which places a signature or thumbprint on each of one's actions, making it recognizably one's own.' We already know that we all have different desires and needs, and our temperament shows us how our behaviour is geared to obtaining these. Here are the descriptions of the four temperaments.

NF Temperament (ENFJ, INFJ, ENFP and INFP)

NFs play a prominent part in our society, as their unique contributions make them stand out. Their needs and aspirations are seldom understood easily, so they may be something of an enigma to the other three temperaments. Their prime need, which is to 'be' rather than to 'do', is tied up with a search for their personal identity, and is complex to explain to those who view the world in a more concrete and material way. Likewise, NFs may have some difficulty in comprehending the values and needs of the other three temperaments.

This search for self continues throughout life, and NFs are frequently found in spiritual and psychological groups, and groups aimed at personal growth. Here, they feel at home as they are among those who are on a similar path. NFs often become therapists as they have an intuitive sense of people's feelings and needs; indeed they may need therapy themselves as they can overload themselves with the troubles of others. It is important to NFs to be genuine and to bring their own contributions to everything they are involved with. Taken to extremes, their striving for their own and others' personal development may cause NFs some unhappiness as they are sensitive to small tensions in relationships. NFs are prepared to invest a lot in most of their relationships, and can be bitterly disappointed if any of them go wrong.

Words are an NF forte, and usually NFs are gifted at communicating and writing. No other temperament has this gift like NFs do, and NFs are highly represented in the communications business. NFs can use words in a personal way that persuades others, and explain things so that they can understand. And NFs communicate that they care, and are interested and concerned with people's personal lives. As writers,

NFs can express how others feel about the significance and meaning of life, and they can be an inspiration to people. Most creative writers and writers of fiction belong to the NF temperament; scientific and technical writers tend to be NTs.

Work that limits NFs to deal only with things rather than people is unlikely to be satisfying. NFs need work that allows them to bring out the best in people, as they are always on the look-out for possibilities in others. NFs are drawn to work in personnel, teaching, counselling, or public relations; they are also attracted to psychology, psychiatry, alternative medicine, the church and other spiritual groups. NFs find the arts – including languages, social sciences and the whole artistic world – more comfortable than technology and the world of commerce. Although not commercially minded, NFs will happily work in the business world provided the work involves people.

NFs are found, too, in a variety of jobs in the theatre, and in radio and television. Where the SP is in these places to perform, NFs are there to communicate. When acting they virtually 'become' the person, taking on his/her identity.

As speakers NFs are gifted, usually having the ability to persuade and convince others. If they are committed to a cause – and most NFs are deeply and profoundly committed to something – they can easily collect followers.

It is not difficult for NFs to help others to be more kind or more humane. But it is hard for them to say 'No' to anything, and NFPs especially need to learn to limit the output of their time and energy. Ideas and projects may have instant appeal to NFs when they are proposed, but as their focus is on the future they may drop these ideas once something else comes along. This can happen with people, too. NFs may give their loyalty, commitment and belief to someone, and then drop them for someone else. The first person may have no idea why they have been dropped.

A partner answers the NF need for romance in their life, and they believe in true and lasting love. Harmony and high standards are important to NFs, and they are idealistic about their relationships. The mundane quality of day-to-day life may let NFs down, and the reality of their relationships disappoint them. One reason for this may be that NFs are not always geared into the practicalities of living in this world. NFs become emotional easily; Es speak out and express their emotions but Is tend to keep their emotions inside themselves.

NFs are generally full of goodwill to others. Most NFs dislike expressing hostility and go out of their way to avoid doing this. For this reason they can defuse tense or disturbed situations by bringing harmony to them.

46

NFs have a strong fantasy life, dreaming of romantic and magical possibilities, and they are able to put much of this into writing – and frequently they do. Is consider some of this so private that it is seldom shown to others. If your writing – or any other work you have put your heart into – is criticized, you are easily discouraged and may not offer your work again.

It is helpful to NFs if they remember to look at situations from a Sensing and Thinking viewpoint. This helps them to be more realistic and logical. There is more about this in Chapter 12.

About 10 per cent of the general population are NFs, and since we have more F females we have more females than males in this group. Again, there are more Es than Is, so we have more ENFJs and ENFPs than INFJs and INFPs.

NT temperament (ENTJ, INTJ, ENTP and INTP)

NTs are governed by their need to understand and explain the universe. At heart they are scientists, bringing a scientific attitude to all that makes up the world. NTs also bring a logical and creative mind to anything they consider, and like to feel they are in control of their lives.

Intelligence is valued by NTs – both in themselves and in others – and they are likely to continue acquiring knowledge throughout their lives. New ideas and concepts, and new ways of tackling things are tucked away in the NT mind. Learning new skills and subjects appeals to NTs, and they usually have some new project on the go. If they are acquiring a new skill, NTs push themselves hard but are seldom satisfied with their achievements: each level of achievement is never enough, NTs then push themselves onto the next level. Being competent and effective at what they do is important to NTs and they are critical of themselves.

NTs live in the future, often at the expense of not being fully in the present. Their minds leap ahead to plan new ways of doing things, and they are excellent strategists and planners. Events and consequences are foreseen, which can be valuable in business. When NTs have ideas they are visualized as having happened, but sometimes NTs may not be aware of the practical details needed for turning these ideas into reality, so they do not necessarily come to fruition. Ps do not mind so much about this, as their need is to generate ideas rather than to work them through step-by-step. Js drive themselves relentlessly to put their ideas into action, and both Js and Ps may on occasions take the wrong steps to achieve something.

Accuracy and precision are valued by NTs, and people look on them as being a bit arrogant and splitting hairs in an argument; any redundancy of words or effort annoys NTs, and they dislike wasted time or effort.

It comes naturally to NTs to group and classify things, but quantifying is harder; assessing how long, for example, a job will take may be more difficult. As their mind is frequently focused on the future NTs may be unaware of the passing of time in the present.

NTs focus on the future, and the desire for progress leads them to excel in science and technology. NTs love solving problems and improving ways of doing things. Working at improving something gives NTs infinitely more pleasure than any amount of leisure. NTs tend to get completely absorbed in whatever they are working on – often neglecting day-to-day social niceties. And they find it hard to relax and have fun, and may feel somewhat awkard on social occasions as they tend not to go in for small talk.

NTs decide what they want to be involved in and make this clear to those around them. Before joining any group NTs need to see demonstrated a logical reason for its existence. Outwardly, NTs are usually calm and controlled, and this is due to their strong sense of reason and willpower.

Maintaining things or businesses usually fails to satisfy NTs as they function best with a problem to solve. When they put forward their ideas, NTs express them precisely and accurately, but may omit to tell others of the important practical steps, assuming they can fill these in. NTs are rarely content with their achievements and push themselves on to achieve more, and any mistakes they make annoy them greatly. NTs believe in justice and fairness.

The shadow side of the NT is SF – the Sensing and Feeling preferences – and these are less developed in the NT. People who are SFs are well aware of the practical requirements in our homes and in our society. They are the ones who care for our actual day-to-day needs, whether this is to help us on with our coat, nurse us when we are ill or to see we have all we need in our material life. These are the things that NTs are less aware of and others may feel NTs are uncaring.

Around 10 per cent of the general population are NTs, and as there are more male Ts there are more male NTs than female. Again, there are more Es than Is, so there are more ENTJs and ENTPs than INTJs and INTPs.

SJ temperament (ESTJ, ISTJ, ESFJ, ISFJ)

We tend to meet this temperament often – at work, in our family and in our social lives. In our society we are conscious of SJs in many areas – in fact our society would not carry on without SJs, as they maintain and look after many of its aspects. SJs are concerned with being useful and doing their duty. They support and believe in most of society's institutions, and are prepared to spend their time seeing that these are functioning well and organized properly. SJs are the most traditional temperament and therefore the most traditional people.

SJs like to belong to society and to be part of it; often they are members of a number of groups and clubs. SJs are willing to take on jobs in the community that other temperaments tend to avoid; jobs involving practical service to others, caretaking, and maintaining, and seeing to small details are tasks usually volunteered for by SJs. SJs are aware of the need to look after the many tasks involved in running organizations and enjoy taking part in these responsibilities. SJs are known as the guardians of our society, since they guard us against adverse events, misfortune and ruin.

SJs act responsibly, and can be relied on to carry out instructions and agreements; rules and regulations, and budgets and reports will be seen to. Much time is devoted to these, the Is being willing to work for hours to check them through meticulously. SJs work hard at whatever they do, and they may take on work that overloads them – out of a feeling of duty.

When it comes to choosing a career, SJs are invariably drawn to work which supports society. Safeguarding our security is important to SJs, and they may go in for insurance, accountancy, law or banking; they are also attracted to teaching, the church, the civil service and a variety of administrative posts – even medicine or social work – especially the care of the old or the young. And being practical, well-organized and thrifty SJs are successful in business and industry, often rising to top executive positions. Knowing names and titles is considered important, and SJs accept and support authority and position.

SJs collect and absorb many detailed facts, and the past is important to them; decisions are based on past experience and information, and SJs are less likely to see future possibilities. Work that other temperaments might consider boring or repetitive will be seen by SJs to be necessary and important – and they will see it is done. If someone else is responsible for a job the SJ is likely to check up on him/her to be certain it is accomplished properly and on time. In community or business groups and clubs SJs are prepared to take on the roles that monitor the details, check the funds, see to the minutes and ensure that plans are carried through. As for the clearing up after events, it is most likely that this, too, is done by SJs.

Time is something actual and concrete for SJs, and they are punctual and good timekeepers, usually having a sense of how long a job will take and planning their time accordingly. With their awareness of the importance of each necessary step in any process, they can become pessimistic, since they are often aware of the things that can go wrong.

Above all, SJs insist on being useful; abstractions and possibilities are of little interest, as they need to see an actual result. SJs are serious people, and as children were generally good pupils at school. The way of life at school suited them, and the SJ would have been in the right place at the right time, well behaved and handing in homework on time.

Our less developed preferences usually indicate areas to which we pay less attention. With the SJs these are likely to be the N and P preferences – the characteristics that look at new ideas and possibilities. SJs are more likely to consider and deal with the facts they know, and less likely to consider concepts and theories which are merely suppositions. It can be helpful and profitable for SJs to listen to other temperaments to get a different angle on projects and situations, and especially to be willing to consider long-term plans and ideas.

Much leisure time is likely to be taken up with commitments in the community, often continuing with what the SJ does at work. Fortunately for society, nature has provided plenty of SJs, and we have around 45 per cent in the general population. Since we have more Es than Is we have more ESTJs and ESFJs than ISTJs and ISFJs.

SP temperament (ESTP, ISTP, ESFP and ISFP)

Someone with the SP temperament group may well not be reading this book! SPs are action-oriented people, valuing their freedom and having little time for theories. They like to be doing something rather than talking about doing it.

Although there are many SPs in our society they tend not to be found in groups in the community like the SJs. Work or leisure that has a strict routine does not attract SPs, and if they find themselves in too organized a structure, may seldom stay long. If the opportunity arises – and SPs are quick to seize it if it does – SPs choose work that provides variety and some excitement. Without this they become bored easily.

Of all the temperaments, SPs live most fully in the present moment, and are acutely conscious of small minute-by-minute changes in the environment. Where many others have difficulty adapting to these changes SPs adapt easily. Those who know SPs look on them as light-hearted, fun, charming and witty. Deep and intimate discussions are not the province of SPs as they can be somewhat perplexed by having to deal with personal feelings and emotions.

For SPs, life is to be lived to the full and enjoyed – SPs have a great capacity for refusing to see or accept a misfortune or calamity. Other temperaments may be flattened by disasters but SPs will rise above these, always believing luck will change and good days lie ahead. The SPs' happy-go-lucky attitude may not be shared by their partners – especially if they are Js. The impulsive nature, which is what governs SP actions, may land them in trouble at times, both at home and at work.

Where SJs tend to conserve and save money, SPs spend freely, often being generous to those around them. If things are going well, SPs may share the benefits with others, but they do not get too down if things turn against them. The five senses of touch, taste, smell, hearing and sight are well developed in SPs, and they are confident in practical living.

Unlike the SJ, who felt at home in school, SPs were frequently unhappy there as school required a more theoretical and disciplined life. Once they had left primary school, SPs may have had little opportunity for active practical learning – which was a pity because SPs learn by doing; Ns learn by hearing and understanding theory, but SPs need to move around and find out how things work in action.

Using tools is something SPs excel at – whether for practical use in the home or garden, or for artistic purposes, or in the construction industry. Machinery holds no terrors for SPs and they are prepared to operate machines with confidence and economy. Once SPs have felt, smelt, tasted, seen or heard how something works, they remember it, and they enjoy the activity involved.

SPs may not be the most punctual of people, and if something better is in the offing they can turn a blind eye to a previous arrangement. This is certain to upset other, more organized types – in particular those who are strong Js. Although SPs can glide easily from project to project – seldom running out of energy if the project interests them – they may not be good timekeepers. Precise hours and minutes are not important to SPs – for them it is more important to be doing what life offers at any given moment.

SPs can act and perform for the benefit of themselves and others. They can operate on both things and people, and can entertain. Similarly, their work needs to have variety and action in it. Entrepreneurs, troubleshooters, surgeons, pilots, entertainers, musicians and all types of artists are frequently from the SP temperament.

SPs are less constrained by duty than other temperaments as they are more playful and easy-going. In business, SPs like fun and excitement, and a crisis can be stimulating. In fact, SPs are often at their best in a crisis, and they work long hours and endure physically uncomfortable situations. When down on their luck, SPs can make use of anything that is available, and they can live happily and frugally. Their entrepreneurial qualities can be used at these times, but once the crisis has become stabilized the SP will lose interest. Many an SP has successfully got a business off the ground and the business has then failed through inattention to maintaining it.

Like the SJs, SPs are inclined to dislike anything abstract; things must be concrete, useful and actually happen; why they happen is of no interest.

As family members SPs are flexible and believe everyone is equal. As a parent, SPs can be unpredictable but easy-going; rather than create a nest for the family they are likely to encourage freedom and independence, letting each member pursue his or her own interests. Family rituals and ceremonies are turned into festivities and frivolities. No other temperament enters so abundantly into celebrations as the SP does, and SPs have a great capacity for enjoying the pleasures of the senses to the full. Any excuse for celebrating an occasion is welcomed by SPs.

The characteristics of N and J are least likely to be developed in SPs: N brings forth ideas and concepts – often abstract ones – and J puts these into action. SPs are more likely to make use of things that exist today than dream up possibilities for tomorrow; and they are more likely to be juggling a number of things around than settling on one of them. At times, however, it might be helpful to take the advice or ask the opinion of a type who is N and J.

There are around 35 per cent SPs in the general population, and equal numbers of males and females. With more Es around we can expect more ESTPs and ESFPs, with fewer ISTPs and ISFPs. In the past years the SP female has had a hard time in our society with little opportunity for her natural talents, but society's attitude is changing and better opportunities are now coming the way of SP females.

Summary

The lists below help us to see the differences in behaviour between the temperaments in similar situations.

Whereas NFs try to provide a comfortable situation for others,
    NTs let us know their boundaries
    SJs gather together in groups
    SPs hunt around for interest.

Whereas NFs become emotional,
    NTs stay calm
    SJs get worried
    SPs get excited.

Whereas NFs look for inspiration and meaning,
    NTs like to gain rational insights
    SJs enjoy rituals and ceremonies
    SPs enjoy festivities and frivolities.

Whereas NFs excel in understanding literature at school,
NTs succeed in science and technology
SJs do well in business studies
SPs learn by doing.

Becoming aware of our temperamental differences gives us an *overall* method of understanding ourselves. It is surprising how satisfying it is when we discover friends, colleagues and family who share our temperament. We find we have much in common with them in our pattern of living, as temperament is at the core of our personality.

The next two chapters tells us about the work we enjoy and how we are likely to behave at work.

6

Personality Conflicts
at Work

Whatever work we are drawn to, all of us want a working lifestyle which brings us satisfaction and happiness. But when we choose our work we may be constrained by our circumstances and our personal situation, and by the social and cultural expectations around us. In spite of these we find that our type and temperament dictate our interests, our abilities and our behaviour, and when we are unable to follow these our working life may be frustrating and unfulfilling.

Few of us have complete freedom to choose the exact work we would like to be doing, but we can use our knowledge of type and temperament to guide us towards a working life that suits us. Most of us need to earn money in paid employment for a good part of our lives, and the work we do and the conditions in which we do this have an immense effect on how happy and successful we are. When our work fits in with our preferences for living we produce our best and feel good. It is as simple as that. And the more our work requires us to use the qualities and characteristics that are in our shadow the more stressed and unhappy we are likely to be. Those around us suffer too, as we are frustrated and present our worst side to them instead of our best. There is more about our shadow in Chapter 12.

As we become more aware of different work patterns we can see why some work comes easily to us and other work is more difficult. We often undervalue the things we do easily, which is unfortunate as this is where we are likely to be most successful. We can recognize, too, that people who act and think differently from us at work may not be deliberately trying to antagonize us; it is more likely that their way of experiencing life is quite different from our way. There are many occasions when they may be just the person we need to help us check on our plans and data, as their opinion is likely to bring greater balance to our decisions and actions.

This chapter concentrates on some of the conflicts that happen at work, and helps us to see how these arise. We look, too, at how some of these can be resolved.

We can start by reminding ourselves about the different preferences as we look briefly at how these affect the needs of everyone at work.

Extraverts Energized by the outer world of people and things; at work they need to act quickly and they bring their ideas into shape by discussion.

Introverts More energized by the inner world of thoughts and reflections; at work they need to think before acting and they need time for quiet reflection.

Sensers Process information through the five senses; they like to do work of a practical nature, using their experience and facts.

INtuitives Process information through patterns and relationships; they like to work at solving problems and changing things.

Thinkers Base their decisions on logic and objectivity; at work they are logical and firm minded with others.

Feelers Base their decisions on personal subjective values; at work they are friendly and personal with others.

Judgers Need work that allows them to be structured, orderly and organized; they like to plan and reach decisions.

Perceivers Prefer work that allows them to be flexible, adaptable and spontaneous; they like to leave things open to change.

We can compare some of the ways in which we go about our work and look at some of the personal situations which arise; this helps us to recognize our differences and to see how we can benefit from these rather than get into conflict.

Extraverts and Introverts

We know that Es like to work with other people, and their energy is generally recharged by having others around them as they do their best work this way. They are quick to think in most situations, and they act fast to get things done. Extraverts are attracted to the outside world, and if they have to work on their own for lengthy periods of time they are likely to have trouble concentrating, as they are drawn to the outside.

Introverts are different and they prefer to work quietly, often on their own, and this is how they produce their best work. They prefer to think things over more slowly, seldom letting others know what they feel until they have finished this process. If their work involves public speaking they may find it difficult to speak fluently without plenty of preparation. Extraverts, who tend to be on the boil and raring to go all the time, expect some steady feedback from the I. An example of how this happens follows.

An advertising agency in London held meetings every week between the four creative personnel to focus on a two-year project they were all working on. Three of them were Es, and the fourth was an I. The Es looked forward to the meeting each week, enjoying each other's company and using the time to bounce ideas off one another. Quick and energetic talk flowed between the three of them. At the end of each meeting all the Es felt elated, and returned to their offices encouraged to press on with their work.

For the I the weekly meeting was a different experience. He, too, enjoyed the exchange of ideas, and when the meeting was over he spent a good deal of his time planning how he could make use of what had been discussed. But during the actual meeting he hardly said a word, and the three Es thought this was because he had nothing to contribute. This was not the case. He had a lot to contribute, but he needed time to consider before he came out with his ideas. Also, as the three Es were talking so much between themselves he hardly got a chance!

When the four of them came to an understanding of their E and I preferences they decided to make a point of providing time for the I to contribute. The Es continued to enjoy their quick exchanges, but one of them would remember to turn to the I from time to time and specifically ask him what he felt about the topic under discussion; if the I was slow to reply the Es learnt not to rush him but to wait. At the end of the meeting they again made sure to ask him if he had anything further he would like to say. After holding their meetings for some months this way the Es said they were amazed at the amount the I contributed, and the I said he valued being given time for this and he felt more part of the meeting. All agreed they got more out of the weekly meeting this way.

Extraverts need other people at work to communicate with. They often work out their ideas and problems by talking to colleagues. If an E is shut up alone in his/her office all day he/she may feel discouraged and depressed, and is likely to look around for someone to have a chat with. After a break and a chat the E feels happy to get back to work.

Introverts generally do their best work on their own – certainly they prefer a quiet atmosphere to a talkative one. At work they can find an E's need to talk both perplexing and annoying. If they find themselves in a noisy office, they do not always know why they are not producing their best work. But when they understand their need for quiet – and are able to obtain this – they are much happier and their work improves.

When we understand that Es and Is have different needs for working environments we can give due importance to these when we do our work.

John, an I accountant working in a large open-plan office, realized his working space was positioned on the way to the tea and coffee machine. Throughout the day colleagues would come past his working space, often in twos and threes, chatting to one another because it was time for a break. If they had to wait their turn they frequently included him in their conversation, disturbing his train of thought. John knew he worked best if he could have long periods undisturbed. He noticed there was an unused working space, tucked away in the far corner. He asked his boss if he could move there, being careful to explain that he would be able to work better. He did move there, and is happier and more productive in his own corner.

For Jennifer, an E, the situation was quite different. She had been in market research for some years before she married. She thought how nice it would be to have time to herself, and with a large house to look after there seemed plenty to do. After a year she found she got depressed spending much of the day on her own, and she felt she would like to return to work part-time. She was fortunate enough to find just the work she wanted locally. A month later she realized why it was she had wanted to return to work: 'I can't believe how much happier I feel,' she said, 'I hadn't realized how much I depended on my colleagues at work. It's not just the work I do, it's being in touch with the other people and those I interview, and generally having someone to talk to. Some of the people I interview tell me quite a bit about their lives, and I really enjoy that.' Jennifer has a better understanding of her E preference now, and has valued her work more since she has recognized it takes her into the outer world.

Extraverts can work better with Is by giving them some personal space and time on their own to work. And when Es talk to Is they need to be sure not to do all the talking, as this gives the I no chance to contribute. Extraverts may need to become good listeners as they learn a lot by doing this. At work Es can also let Is know of matters to be discussed in advance, perhaps in writing, as this gives the I time to consider the matter.

Introverts can work better with Es by learning to speak out when necessary. And Is need to take their chance in discussions as they may not get many! For them it is a case of deliberately bringing out their E when they need to make a point, knowing they can return to their I when this is done. It is important that Is let their work colleagues know they need peace and quiet in which to do their best work; in a large office Is are likely to be working with a number of Es who are probably unaware of this.

All business environments can benefit when they give some consideration to the needs of their Es and Is.

Sensers and iNtuitives

Our E and I preference usually becomes apparent as we work with other people over a period of time. But with our S and N preferences this is not always so noticeable. If it is possible for us to know our own preference and the preference of those we work with closely, we can avoid a lot of conflict. We can work better together and have more realistic expectations of one another.

At work Ss take in information about things in a definite and measurable way. They notice specific parts and details, and they go to the beginning of things and look for procedures and instructions. They like things which are tangible, and work steadily step-by-step, usually having a good sense of time. If they do not look beyond the present they may not be aware of how the situation might be in the future. They prefer working with things they understand than with possibilities, and they are good at dealing with facts.

INtuitives are quite different at work as they look for links and patterns in things. They notice the whole rather than the details, and look at how things relate to one another rather than looking at the specific parts and pieces. Often they follow their hunch, wanting to change things and suggesting new ways of doing this. They prefer to be engaged in working on new projects and problems than seeing to the maintenance of routine necessities. In looking forward to the future they may neglect the important details of the present. Here is an example of the way in which Ss and Ns can see the same situation.

Two friends, one an S and the other an N, were asked to join a charity committee that ran a group of sheltered homes for the elderly. John is an S, Tom is an N. For six months they attended monthly committee meetings, usually travelling home together. John, the S, seemed quite happy with the way the committee was run. He felt the topics they discussed and the attention given to the small details of the day-to-day running of the homes was good. Tom, an N, felt otherwise. After several meetings, which consisted of practical details relating to the homes, such as the construction of the buildings, the kitchen facilities, the safety of the roof and the staff procedures, Tom felt the meetings were tedious and frustrating.

As they were going home one evening they started to discuss their different feelings about the content of the committee meetings. Tom burst out with his frustration: 'In six months we haven't once talked about our plans for the future or ways in which we could make improvements in the homes. All we've done is endlessly discuss petty details. A sub-committee could see to these, leaving us to get on with the real work of making plans to improve the homes.' 'How can you feel that?' replied John in amazement, 'Why, it's an excellent committee. The chairman is meticulous over details and sees these are brought up at every meeting. We are all given our chance to speak on each topic, so everything is covered thoroughly. Also, all the important matters like safety, building regulations and staff procedures are brought up every month.' 'That's just it,' said Tom, 'We're so concerned with the minute details of keeping the homes going at a practical level that we never have time to get on to the important matters of making alterations and developing the homes.' 'The practical day-to-day running of the homes *is* important, in fact it's the most important of all,' replied John.

We can see that John and Tom consider different things to be important. Both of their views are needed. Tom is right in saying that if all the committee time is taken up with small practical details there is none left for future plans and development. Equally, John is right in placing importance on the day-to-day running of the homes, as they would not continue to function without this attention. In this case the company has an S chairman, and this explains why the committee is run on S lines. John, as another S, feels comfortable with this, whereas Tom, as an N, feels less comfortable.

John saw Tom's point and suggested he bring up his ideas at the next meeting. Others on the committee saw the value of including time to consider future plans and possibilities, and the committee asked Tom to put forward some of his ideas at the next meeting, and agreed to spend some time each month discussing these. Tom felt much happier about this.

Sensers and iNtuitives can have major misunderstandings at work unless they are aware of each other's preference for absorbing information. Here is another example:

Each year one of our city councils is responsible for putting on a summer exhibition. The preparation for the exhibition takes about two months and responsibility for this is usually given to two of their senior employees. This year one of them was away on maternity leave, so a substitute was found.

Margaret, who had prepared the exhibition for three previous years, had worked happily during this time with Mary, who was now on maternity leave. Margaret and Mary were both Ss, in fact both were ISFJs. Preparing the exhibition together had been something they had both enjoyed working on.

When Margaret heard that Jackie was to work with her she wondered how they would manage. Jackie was known for always wanting to change things; she was rarely content to let things be. Jackie was an N. When they started their work Margaret spent a morning having a look at what they had done the previous year. She then told Jackie she felt they should set the exhibits out in the same way as last year, and the programme of events could also be kept exactly the same.

Jackie – as was expected – was appalled. As she read through last year's programme she was mentally making alterations. 'Let's try something different this year,' she said, 'We could switch round some of the events. And let's move the venue to another part of town. By the new arcade would be a good place.' 'But why?' replied Margaret, 'If something works well it seems sensible to keep it that way. Why alter something for no reason?' 'There *is* a reason,' said Jackie, 'By putting it in a new place people will notice it, and if we change the events round it gives some variety to the exhibition. No one wants to go to the same old thing as last year.'

But Margaret thought otherwise. The exhibition had been a success the past three years. Being an S, and also SJ temperament, she believed that if a formula worked it was best to repeat it. She was also against changing the venue to another part of the city, as she felt that after three years people would expect the exhibition to be where it had always been; she felt that changing the venue would muddle people.

Jackie, who had not been involved in the previous exhibitions, saw the opportunity to create something different in the city. Her mind scanned over the various events during the past few years and she tried to come up with something different. INtuitives tend to look for new ways of doing things.

Margaret and Jackie spent a lot of time arguing about how the exhibition should be best organized. Neither could see the other's point of view. If they had been aware of both their preferences for absorbing information they would have had a better understanding of the other's way of thinking. In the end they agreed on a compromise. The venue and the display of exhibits would remain the same and Margaret would be responsible for all these arrangements. But Jackie was given charge of re-arranging the events during the exhibition, which gave scope for her N.

Margaret and Jackie might have still come to the same agreement if they had already known each other's preference for S or N, but it could have been with less argument and with a view to the importance of considering the other's opinion.

Sensers and iNtuitives can also interpret and focus on written material differently. Here is an example of this.

Two directors of a building company, one an S and the other an N, were handed a report on the staff canteen and asked to give their comments at a meeting later that day.

The S picked out two specific items relating to kitchen safety and staff procedure. He drew attention to the need for a further safety check on the cooker and the importance of placing the instructions for kitchen staff where they could be clearly seen. While he was talking about these the N was impatiently waiting his turn. When asked for his comments he said he felt the report 'in general' was good but the company needed to think up better ways of making use of their employees. One suggestion he had for doing this would be for everyone to help themselves to food at lunch rather than using one of the staff at the canteen. This way the company could cut down on the kitchen staff and save some money.

The S director looked for practical details in the report, and then focused his attention on these, ending in making two suggestions that contributed to the health and safety of the kitchen staff. The N, who was also an NT and therefore disliked waste of personnel, skipped the practical details and looked at the general picture for what might be done in the way of improvement. We can notice that the S focused on the details of the report, especially the practical details, but the N focused on the report as a whole and his suggestions for improvement came out of this. Neither of them paid much attention to the items the other felt to be important. Both contributions were needed, but they were different. It is unlikely that either of them could have made the other's suggestions.

In this case we see the value of having an S and an N director, provided that both recognize the contribution the other can bring. Between them they covered the report more thoroughly, and both were able to use their abilities for the benefit of their company.

The problems of promotion perplex many of us. These often involve our S and N preferences. As we climb the ladder at work our responsibilities change. Work that was largely S work, for example, may change to needing more of our N. Many people cannot understand why they have more difficulty once they are promoted. When we start a job we need to look ahead to see what the job may become in the future.

Sensers can work better with Ns if they are prepared to listen to their ideas to see if these can work. Often the Ss are the ones who can put the ideas into action. But Ss can get fixated on single items and facts, and they need to see how these fit into the business as a whole. It can help Ss if they try to look ahead.

INtuitives can work better with Ss if they are prepared to check out their ideas and schemes with them, as the Ss can let them know if these can work out in a practical manner. INtuitives need to give attention to the actual details of the present, as they easily forget these by getting carried away by their thoughts for the future. INtuitives may need to improve their sense of time, which may be poor because Ns are often not in the present moment.

Thinkers and Feelers

When we include the viewpoints of both Ts and Fs at work we bring more balance to our business and work decisions. Thinkers, who have the advantage of being able to stand outside situations, use their heads to be analytical and logical, and they can see flaws and be good critics. Often they can present material to others by writing clear papers and documents. These are all important qualities in promoting, assessing and running many businesses.

But Fs have equally important advantages. They are gifted at dealing with people and at understanding them, and are usually good communicators. People's feelings and their relationships are important to Fs, and they make a big contribution towards keeping staff happy and harmonious. Thinkers may be able to present an idea or report on paper better, but Fs are more likely to be able to persuade people to accept the contents of the idea or report. They have a way of telling people about things that shows up the benefits.

At work Ts tend to be firm and impersonal and they feel they are working for their company; Fs tend to be more yielding and personal and feel they are working for – and with – the people in their company. At times these attitudes may conflict. Here is an example:

A medium-sized manufacturing company was forced to close one of its plants, and this meant a redundancy operation was going on. The two personnel managers met to finalize the terms and conditions of the 30 personnel involved. John and Peter's day-to-day work generally kept them apart, but today they met to sort out the details of the redundancy. John is a T and Peter is an F.

'There's only one thing to do' said John, 'and that is to arrange a meeting for all 30 to attend, and not to beat about the bush, but just to tell them straight. At the same time we can let them know about the redundancy terms. Do you agree with this, Peter?' Peter hesitated – Peter is an I as well as an F – and he did not appear to be too happy. 'To suddenly spring it on everyone in a group meeting seems a bit harsh, John. It really will be a bombshell for most people, can you imagine those with families to support having to go home and tell them?' 'Peter, I know it's hard, I was made redundant once myself many years ago, and it's tough. When it happened to me I had to grin and bear it, and get going to look for something else. I can't do anything for any of these people, we've just got to get rid of them, and I've got to get on with my day-to-day work for the company.'

John's first consideration was to get the redundancy over quickly so that he could continue to do his best work for the company. Peter's first consideration was for those who were being made redundant. Peter continued: 'I do feel we should see each person privately and break this to them gently, enquiring if there are things we could do to help them find new work. We must give each of them a reference and suggest other companies to approach. Many of these people have been with us for years, and they deserve some support and care from us.' 'We just haven't got the time, Peter,' said John, 'Do you want us to spend our days looking after people who are not going to be working for us in future? If so, the company will suffer. How will our work get done?'

The conversation went on. It became clear that the two men had quite different ideas on how to manage the redundancy. In the end John came up with the suggestion that he would continue with the day-to-day personnel work for the company while Peter took over the management of the redundancy operation. This way John felt he was continuing working for the company, and Peter was able to use his understanding of people to give time and personal attention to everyone who was made redundant. Both were making use of their relevant T and F preferences.

Here is another instance of T and F differences:

A paper manufacturing company depends on its computer department for current information. One Thursday afternoon the main computer broke down, leaving all personnel without the information they needed to continue business. The department worked all day Friday and finally located the fault. It would need two of the analysts to work all weekend to put things right for Monday. Neville (a T), in charge of the computer department, informed Richard (an F), the director responsible for distribution.

'We've located the fault, and we're putting Jonathan and Anne on overtime so we should have everything back to normal by Monday morning', reported Neville. 'It means they'll both have to work all weekend, but it will be worth it.'

'That's good news', replied Richard. 'It doesn't sound as if it will be a very good weekend for Jonathan and Anne though, it's good of them to do this. You'll be putting them on double pay, of course.'

'Certainly not, and it's not good of them', responded Neville. 'It's in their contracts to be available for overtime at weekends.'

'I know,' said Richard, 'but it will be a long slog, and I feel they deserve double pay. I feel they should have Monday off, too, and we should let them charge up a good meal each day. It will give them a break and help them to work better.'

'Rubbish', exploded Neville. 'This is all part of their work contract and I shall expect them in on Monday as usual.'

Neville expressed a T view when he pointed out that weekend work was part of the contract. He was more concerned with getting the work done for the company than for the personal situation of Jonathan and Anne.

Richard expressed an F view when he considered the personal situation of Jonathan and Anne. He thought about their need to eat and to have a break. He also felt they were likely to be tired by Monday morning and would deserve a day off before starting another week.

Both points of view needed to be considered. Neither Neville nor Richard was likely to change their attitude, but if both had been aware of each other's T and F preferences they could have taken this into account when they made a decision.

One of the commonest grouses between Ts and Fs at work has to do with minor day-to-day communications. Small jobs around the office are just small jobs around the office for Ts; but for Fs they are an opportunity for being pleasant to people, and they like it when people are pleasant in return – perhaps a smile or an affable thankyou. This shows us the difference between the Ts' more impersonal way of relating to others and the Fs' more personal way. Thinkers say they are perplexed as to why Fs need to be 'smiling all the time' at work and Fs say they wonder why Ts are so cold and unemotional.

Thinkers can work better with Fs if they pay attention to how issues at work affect the staff, and not just the business, and if they make an effort to see that people's feelings are not hurt. Thinkers can unwittingly hurt people's feelings at work. They have more difficulty expressing their emotions, and if they can do this calmly it helps people to know how they feel.

Feelers can work better with Ts when they try not to take things personally. Feelers personalize most things, even feeling involved with situations which they are not responsible for. If Fs can speak out over issues, even if they are in disagreement with someone, this clears the air and makes it easier for everyone to be open.

Differences between Ts and Fs are usually easier to come to terms with than other differences, as Ts can see the value of an F's point of view, and Fs can do the same with a T's point of view. When both can express how they feel it is easier to make decisions that take both views into consideration.

Judgers and Perceivers

We know that Js prefer a lifestyle which is *more* organized, planned and structured, and Ps prefer a lifestyle which is *less* organized, planned and structured. It is not difficult to see these differences at work, and this is where they cause some of the greatest conflicts.

Whatever type of work is involved, Js and Ps set about it in different ways. Judgers invariably want to get the job done, and usually set off to do this as soon as they can.

Unless they can see a good reason to delay doing a job, Js feel happier once it is completed, and they make plans and keep to them. Once Js are in action it is hard to stop them or to change their minds – even if information or circumstances alter – as they are unlikely to be open to new input. Extravert judgers may possibly make up their minds too fast, and start putting things into action too quickly.

Perceivers set about their work in a different way. When they have a job to do they like to gather in as much information about it as they can, and some of them like to delay finishing the job until as late as possible. They like to be flexible as they work, and leave things open to adapt as they go along. If the deadline for completing the job is well ahead they may not produce much tangible work until near the deadline. Sometimes there is a mad rush to get the job finished!

The real clashes between Js and Ps at work come from the Js' urgency to get something completed and the Ps' desire to leave the work open and flexible. Judgers experience great anxiety when they cannot get Ps to complete things. Perceivers feel bound and frustrated when Js are constantly pressing them to finish something. Here is an example of this:

An interior design company was working on a brief for one of their important clients. The job involved designing an extension to the head office, and Geoff and Marianne were given joint responsibility for it. They were given a month in which to produce the finished plans. Geoff and Marianne knew each other through the office but had never worked together on a specific job before. Both were pleased to have been chosen for this important contract.

When they met over coffee they discussed a variety of ways in which they might set about the project. Both of them were Ns, so ideas flowed happily between them. An hour later Geoff – a strong J – had another meeting, so he got out his notebook and suggested they sort out what each of them would do during the next week.

But Marianne wanted to leave her options open rather than be pinned down too early in the project. She said, 'I'll wander round to the library and see what I can turn up, and I'll keep you in touch with things as they emerge. There's no hurry to do anything yet and we can switch our ideas around as we go along.' We can guess from Marianne's words that she is speaking more as a P than as a J.

Geoff was appalled. He had thought they were discussing ideas in order to act on them in the coming week; that way they would have the bones of the project worked out in a week's time, and could then start putting these into action. He wanted to get something specific down in writing so that he could make a start with his work. Marianne's easy-going attitude made him feel unsettled, as he needed something definite to start working on. Also, as a J, he was anxious to be on time for his next meeting. After forcibly expressing his amazement at her attitude he collected his things and dashed off. In the evening when Geoff looked back on the day he felt he had made no progress with the project. He could not understand why, after spending such a fruitful time with Marianne, he could not get her to take specific action on their ideas.

Marianne was also perplexed. What on earth had got into Geoff to make him so irate at the end of their meeting? She, too, felt they had had a good meeting and had covered a lot of ground in talking through the project. It seemed that Geoff wanted to put something definite down on paper, and he was pressing her to do the same.

How ridiculous of him! No one would be doing anything definite about the project until the final week; they needed as much time as they could get to find out a lot of things *before* they could put the project together.

Geoff and Marianne were both committed to the project, but they had different ways of going about it. Geoff, as a J, needed to make a start as soon as he could. He wanted to see something tangible on paper, and he would then build on this to complete his share of the project. He liked to have control of his work and to know that he was on schedule.

Marianne worked in a different way. She was excited by the project, and wanted to follow-up a mass of relevant information. She liked to find out as much as she could before committing herself to anything definite. Often she left finalizing things until the last minute and would have to work late to get everything done. She would have preferred not to rush things at the end but that was the way it always seemed to happen. Generally it did not bother her too much but she could see it sometimes bothered other people.

Throughout the month they worked on their project Geoff and Marianne both felt stressed; they never quite got things together at the same time. Geoff was constantly pressing Marianne to come up with her final work, and Marianne was constantly warding Geoff off.

Geoff and Marianne had no understanding about J and P lifestyles. Their needs – Geoff's for moving to completion and Marianne's for leaving things open to change – were in conflict. If both could have understood the other's way of working, their expectations of one another would have been more realistic. Marianne could have used her abilities to gather ideas and possibilities, but she would have understood Geoff's need to get these ordered and completed in good time; and Geoff could have made a start on something definite, but been willing to make some alterations if something better came along.

Another example of how Js and Ps go about their work is shown in this example about a food company.

The data processing manager of the company was in charge of a department of eight. He had an assistant manager under him, with whom he worked closely. Jim, the manager, is a J. His assistant manager, Oliver, is a P.

Every morning Jim and Oliver meet to check over the day's work for the department. They agree what needs to be done, and Oliver is then responsible for delegating the work to the remaining six employees.

At the end of the day Jim can never understand why the work is seldom completed. Some days are better than others, but on bad days much of the work remains incomplete. At times Jim stays on late to make sure important data is available to the company for the following morning. Finally he tackles Oliver about this, and finds that as the department receives new requests throughout the day Oliver instructs the team to deal with these before completing the pre-arranged day's work. As a result some of the work allocated for the day never gets done, and other departments in the company were complaining.

Oliver, as a P, likes to deal with things as they come up. Each time there is a new request to the department Oliver gives this priority – that is until there is another request, and then this becomes the priority. He spends his day bringing new work to the other six employees. It is easy to see that as more work comes in as the day goes on the original work goes to the bottom of the pile!

Jim is cross and insists that the day's work, which he and Oliver plan each morning, should be carried through as arranged. They do this for a week, and find this does not work either. Although the work planned for each day is completed, none of the new work that arrives throughout the day is ever started. Some of this work needs priority as other departments are complaining that they are not able to get at urgent information.

After Jim and Oliver become aware of their J and P preferences they both try to use these in more positive ways. It is agreed between them that Oliver will allow the day's work to be carried out without interruption until lunchtime. After lunch he will re-programme the rest of the day, taking into account the new work that has come in. If anything comes in later in the afternoon that he considers urgent, then he will ask Jim what they should do. This method worked very much better. After they explained their new method to the other departments the complaints stopped.

One of the most frequent niggles between Js and Ps at work is to do with punctuality and time. When Js arrange a time for doing something or to meet someone they make a point of arriving promptly, and expect everyone else to do the same. A meeting scheduled for 10.00 am is expected to start not later than 10.02. If people wander in around 10.05 or even later Js feel their time is being wasted. Judgers, especially TJs, are good time managers, as they are hard to deflect from the task in hand.

Perceivers have a different attitude to time, and this is evident at work. Times of meetings or times when things are due to start are usually when Ps start to think about getting ready or getting there. If they are close by and there is little preparation to be done they may arrive in time. If they are some way away or have left the preparation until the last minute they may be late, sometimes very late.

Here is another example of J and P in conflict at work:

> Sue and Janice, who work in a management training college, attend a meeting once a month which is chaired by Janice's boss, Steven. Janice and her boss are both Js, and Janice is well aware of the importance Steven places on punctuality. Steven has always gone to the meeting in his car with one of the other directors, and Janice and Sue have always gone in Sue's car. Sue is a P who tends to run late throughout the day, and Sue and Janice seldom arrive on time for the meeting, due to Sue rarely being ready to leave on time. Sue is unperturbed at arriving late, but Janice feels embarrassed and ashamed – especially as she knows the value Steven places on punctuality. After several months of arriving late for this meeting Janice speaks to Steven about this, and he agrees she can have a lift in his car. Janice feels much better, but Sue feels Janice is making a fuss about nothing.

If Js are prepared to accept the input of new information as their work progresses they can work better with Ps. And if Js are willing to look at more options before they make decisions this helps them make a more balanced final decision. Perceivers appreciate it when Js are not so rigid and unbendable. Provided Js can come to agreement with Ps as to the time when work will be produced Js can try not to nag the Ps.

Perceivers can work better with Js if they produce their work on time and keep to deadlines. If Ps break their word about producing work or fulfilling their commitments Js quickly lose their patience and trust in them. If Js feel they cannot rely on Ps they may speak disparagingly about them and try to avoid working with them. When Ps agree times and meetings with Js they should keep to these and not mess the Js about. Perceivers are inclined to have too many projects on the go, and can meet deadlines easier by putting their concentration to one or two things at a time.

This chapter has given us an idea of some of the conflicts that arise at work, and how we can avoid some of these with our understanding of type. The next chapter looks at type in a wider context, and at how our temperament affects our needs and behaviour.

7

Finding Satisfaction:
Type and Work

Let's look more specifically at some of the ways in which each type finds satisfaction at work, and some of the areas of work that are most likely to prove successful for us.

Of course we can be happy and successful in many jobs, provided we can find ways of using our natural pattern of living and our abilities in them. We can also find it helpful to read the information about our opposite type. An ESTJ type, for instance, can read about an INFP type, and vice versa. This gives us added information about ourselves, as it often describes some of the things we find difficult, and this can help us to avoid these things.

Type and work satisfaction

ENFJ

Energized by the outer world; processes information through patterns and relationships; decides by personal subjective values; works best with structure and order.

It is important for ENFJs to have personal contact with people in their work, and they have excellent communication skills. ENFJs are enthusiastic in helping people make the best of themselves, and they do well with work in the media and public relations. They also succeed in teaching, sales and the helping professions, and may be drawn to the church. ENFJs make lots of contacts and their enthusiasm makes them popular as managers and consultants; if work involves leading groups this makes use of their friendly organizational skills. ENFJs are supportive to colleagues and enthusiastic over projects, preferring to work in an orderly fashion. Work that is purely practical or work that leaves them on their own for long makes ENFJs depressed.

If they take care not to slip up on omitting practical details in a project and try to look at situations from an objective view this can help ENFJs.

INFJ

Energized by the inner world; processes information through patterns and relationships; decides by personal subjective values; works best with structure and order.

Quiet, conscientious and spiritually inclined, INFJs have an original mind and need to make use of this for others. Even though it taxes them, they enter into the troubles of those around them, and INFJs have a deep and almost uncanny way of understanding people's feelings. Drawing out the individuality of each person appeals to INFJs, and caring for people's emotional needs through personal therapy or teaching provides this outlet. Often, INFJs are gifted at languages and research work. If their work is creative, INFJs work well alone and are good at following through on projects. INFJs can inspire others to do their best. INFJs do things in an organized manner and are reliable. Work like the transport and building trades that is centred in the concrete hurly-burly of the world is unlikely to suit this type.

If they take care to be aware of what is happening around them in practical terms, and try to speak out assertively, this can help INFJs.

ENFP

Energized by the outer world; processes information through patterns and relationships; decides by personal subjective values; works best with flexibility and adaptability

Ingenious, enthusiastic and outgoing, ENFPs have great personal charm and can be successful at a variety of jobs. ENFPs are quick to see the possibilities of new ideas and projects, and are outstanding at initiating these and persuading people to support them. ENFPs are lively and entertaining, and their energy infectious. This also makes them successful in advertising, sales work, acting and writing. Most ENFPs need change and variety and regularly move on in their work. Journalism suits ENFPs as this allows them to be constantly involved with new things. ENFPs are less suited to work that ties them down to too many routine details; they find it hard to concentrate on these, become bored and let practicalities slip their minds.

They should take care not to take on too many commitments, and make more time to see to the details of completing current work.

INFP

Energized by the inner world; processes information through patterns and relationships; decides by personal subjective values; works best with flexibility and adaptability.

Much of an INFP may be hidden from others at work as s/he is unlikely to express her/his feelings until s/he knows someone well. INFPs can turn their talents to many jobs, but find more satisfaction from work that allows them to use their creativity and personal qualities. Often

71

INFPs excel in languages, art, music and research – bringing enthusiasm and loyalty to their work. As bosses, INFPs encourage co-operation and flexibility. Work which has a spiritual impact is attractive. Practical and repetitive mundane work does not satisfy INFPs: they need to contribute at a personal level, and psychology, counselling and educational work may be of more interest than business. If INFPs find themselves in charge of a business where they have to monitor the detailed work of others they will find this exhausting.

If INFPs take care not to overload themselves with other people's emotions, or to get side-tracked on issues which prevent them from following through in completing important tasks, this will be of benefit.

ENTJ

Energized by the outer world; processes information through patterns and relationships; decides with logic and objectivity; works best with structure and order.

ENTJs need work that allows them to get their teeth into new projects. They are at their best when planning ahead and forecasting for a business, and good at taking those plans into action. ENTJs make capable executives, managers and consultants being successful in reducing inefficiency and time wasting. ENTJs like to be in control and speak out clearly and forcibly when they see the need. Any work associated with science is attractive. ENTJs need work that makes use of their strongly creative drive, and tasks that involve practical day-to-day maintenance tends to frustrate them. Work that alters from day to day according to the whims of the business or client is unlikely to suit ENTJs, as they work better when their plans are not broken into.

ENTJs should take care not to act on things too quickly, and to try to make sure they are co-operative and consider people's feelings.

INTJ

Energized by the inner world; processes information through patterns and relationships; decides with logic and objectivity; works best with structure and order.

INTJs have a creative mind which can be used to bring forward thinking and originality to business and other projects. INTJs are also good at planning and organizing these ideas into action. Their abilities may not be recognized as they may be seen as aloof by others, and they are happier working on their own than as part of a team. INTJs may be drawn to a legal or scientific career, to teaching in higher education or research. INTJs often have good ideas to start and run their own businesses, but may fall down on seeing to the practical details. At work, INTJs are independent, logical and determined. They may work with computers or in medicine if this involves research and analysis.

If their work constantly requires them to be warm and outgoing with the general public this drains INTJs. They should try to check out whether their ideas are practical with others, and not be stubborn about the feedback.

ENTP

Energized by the outer world; processes information through patterns and relationships; decides with logic and objectivity; works best with flexibility and adaptability.

ENTPs need work that provides variety as they are quick and resourceful, and can turn their hands to many things. ENTPs can be entrepreneurs as they are a constant source of ideas. Work that uses their ideas to improve or start a business suits them, but once these ideas get off the ground ENTPs prefer someone else to carry on looking after the business. If they are interested in the product or service, ENTPs are gifted in marketing and sales. ENTPs need work that challenges them and holds their attention, such as public relations, journalism and engineering. ENTPs need colleagues that appreciate their outgoing, talkative and logical manner. The theatre may attract them. No routine practical work interests ENTPs for long, as they need change and variety.

ENTPs should take care not to dash off to the next thing before completing the tasks in hand, and be sure to show appreciation to those who support them.

INTP

Energized by the inner world; processes information through patterns and relationships; decides with logic and objectivity; works best with flexibility and adaptability.

INTPs are reserved and do not generally share their thoughts with those around them. Consequently, many people may not be aware of their complex, adaptable and creative minds. It may not be easy for INTPs to find work that makes use of their unusual intellectual and scientific abilities, but they work well with computer systems, or researching ideas for a project. Ideas are likely to be abstract and contain intellectual insight, but they find the practicalities of carrying out these ideas less interesting. Unless someone else does this INTP ideas may be lost. INTPs do their best work when they are left alone to work quietly, and they are quick and logical at picking out inconsistencies. INTPs are unlikely to commit themselves to routine work that is repetitive and uncreative as they find this frustrating.

INTPs should take care to present their ideas to colleagues in a practical way, and to remember to carry out their current responsibilities.

ESTJ

Energized by the outer world; comfortable using the five senses; decides with logic and objectivity; works best with structure and order.

ESTJs are capable, practical and well rooted in the realistic world of business. Their excellent organizational qualities and commercial aptitude are apparent to those around them, and they frequently rise to the top in management, possibly becoming consultants. ESTJs make good administrators of practical matters in government and military institutions. It is usual for ESTJs to be outspoken, talkative and logical with colleagues. They know what is going on, and they make sure that everyone is doing their bit. ESTJs need practical work that can be tackled step-by-step to produce results, and are likely to have little patience with a work environment that is disorganized or deals with airy-fairy ideas. If an ESTJ goes into medicine it is likely to be in general practice, surgery or obstetrics.

ESTJs should take care to consider the feelings of people they are involved with, and to listen to other people's points of view.

ISTJ

Energized by the inner world; comfortable using the five senses; decides with logic and objectivity; works best with structure and order.

ISTJs tackle their work seriously in a matter-of-fact and orderly manner, placing importance on reading instructions and procedures. Practical and measurable things are their forte, making ISTJs successful in banking, insurance, accountancy and similar businesses. They make good supervisors and administrators at schools, factories and government institutions. Dentists are often ISTJs. Like the ESTJ, ISTJs prefer dealing with figures and practical matters to handling people's emotions. Others may see ISTJs as somewhat duty-bound and impersonal and may not value their dependability in seeing to small details. ISTJs can be relied on to check facts in a quiet, thorough and methodical manner. Work that requires imagination or ideas for the future is likely to be extremely difficult for ISTJs.

ISTJs should take care to consider other people's ideas and feelings, and not to become too rigid and inflexible.

ESFJ

Energized by the outer world; comfortable using the five senses;

decides by personal subjective values; works best with structure and order.

Very sociable, friendly and warm-hearted, ESFJs are best employed in outgoing practical service to others. They are aware of the needs of those around them, sympathetic to those in trouble and good at bringing harmony into the workplace. Nursing and practical medical work is attractive. Our basic requirements of warmth, clothing, health, food and housing are of concern to ESFJs, and when any of these are lacking they are quick to notice. This involvement with human needs is likely to attract ESFJs to work for any of the established institutions, and they do this in an organized, loyal and conscientious way. ESFJs may work, too, for their community – perhaps helping their local school or medical practice, which they do willingly, even if the work is unpaid. Theoretical work holds little interest for ESFJs as they need to be doing something rather than thinking about it. Teaching at primary level suits ESFJs.

ESFJs should take care not to avoid conflict, and try to listen to others carefully and objectively.

ISFJ

Energized by the inner world; comfortable using the five senses; decides by personal subjective values; works best with structure and order.

ISFJs are happiest in work that is of practical service to others, and they provide this quietly, painstakingly and conscientiously – often giving support behind the scenes. Like ESFJs, ISFJs are likely to work in fields related to clothing, health, food or housing. Medical and clerical work suits ISFJs, and they are quiet but friendly in dealing with people. Teaching small children suits ISFJs. ISFJs do not take easily to up-front leadership. If they work in an office, ISFJs are observant of small jobs that need doing, and often offer to do them. They are good at providing customer service. It is not unusual for ISFJs to stay late at work, or to work unpaid, and they may be taken advantage of. Theories hold little interest for ISFJs; they prefer to be doing something.

ISFJs should take care to put forward their own accomplishments, and to be more outspoken and direct.

ESTP

Energized by the outer world; comfortable using the five senses; decides with logic and objectivity; works best with flexibility and adaptability.

ESTPs are good at using their hands to do practical things, and also at working with anything mechanical. ESTPs can be outstanding entrepreneurs in business as they are quick to spot an opportunity and see how this can be turned to advantage. ESTPs are alert to changing situations and can act fast and get results; they are also good at getting people together to negotiate if a project needs this. Attracted to work that involves machines that move, ESTPs enjoy the construction industry and travel. In relating to people at work, ESTPs are down-to-earth and logical, but can be persuasive. As they are able to be spontaneous and versatile at work, ESTPs need excitement and variety – or they lose interest in carrying projects through. Work like one-to-one counselling or solitary academic work is less suitable for ESTPs as they like to be out and about in the world.

ESTPs should take care to look ahead to the consequences of their present actions, and make sure that they do not walk over other people.

ISTP

Energized by the inner world; comfortable using the five senses; decides with logic and objectivity; works best with flexibility and adaptability.

ISTPs are at ease in living and moving around our practical world. They often do well in commerce and if their work requires flexibility and change ISTPs thrive on it. ISTPs have the ability to be detached from issues, viewing them as an onlooker. They are mechanically minded and make good anaesthetists. ISTPs enjoy the excitement of crises at work; they are quick to see what is needed and act accordingly. Making decisions as they go along comes easily to ESTPs, and colleagues may see them as cool and detached. Aspects of teaching and the caring professions that require warm empathy may not suit ISTPs. ISTPs are likely to be happier dealing with things than with people.

ISTPs should take care not to cut too many corners, and be willing to make goals and plan towards them.

ESFP

Energized by the outer world; comfortable using the five senses; decides by personal subjective values; works best with flexibility and adaptability.

Public relations make use of the ESFPs' easy-going, talkative and practical manner. Seldom at a loss in any situation, ESFPs can be relied on to say something to put people at their ease. Full of common sense and friendliness, ESFPs can be most persuasive and a major asset to any sales force. ESFPs are prepared to attempt most things, and enjoy sport and make good coaches, but their work needs to be active rather than theoretical. ESFPs can cope with many projects at once, and being vivacious and tolerant get a lot of fun from the social side of work.

If their work demands that they work alone for long periods they are unhappy, and work that requires abstract reasoning holds little interest.

ESFPs should take care not to leap into things without considering the consequences, and make sure that they complete the tasks they are responsible for before socializing.

ISFP

Energized by the inner world; comfortable using the five senses; decides by personal subjective values; works best with flexibility and adaptability.

Although ISFPs may have business abilities, their modesty and gentle manner prevent them from pushing themselves forward, and they may get overlooked or find themselves in unpaid work. Their talents can be useful in the areas of medicine or dentistry. They can be charmingly persuasive on behalf of others, which makes ISFPs good salespersons. More often ISFPs are behind the scenes working at practical jobs requiring sympathy and service to people – possibly being in the customer service department. ISFPs often have artistic talents, and their feelings may be expressed more through the work they do than in speech. ISFPs are often good at caring for children and animals as they are always aware of the needs of the moment. Managerial work that puts them in charge as the boss or leader does not usually suit ISFPs as they prefer to be more persuasive than directive.

ISFPs should take care to look ahead to the wider consequences of the future, and to assess information in a more objective manner.

Type in organizations

If we work with other people our work is likely to be part of an organization. Organizations are groups of people, and when these are sizeable they are complex to manage and facilitate. They have a purpose – this may be productive, it may be to provide a service, it could be a distribution industry, or something else besides. What is important is that the aims and intentions of the business are clarified. It is then possible for us to sort out what each member of staff is needed for. With this knowledge we are able to have a reasonable idea of which preferences are needed to carry out the work involved, and if we can match these we find our work force becomes happier and more successful. With large organizations this becomes quite complex, but even large organizations divide into smaller groups of departments and teams.

Another aspect of most organizations is that they tend towards a dominant group type, and we find this by seeing which preferences dominate the organization. We look to see if we have more Es or Is, more Ss or Ns etc. As an example we can take a small business with ten staff, and assume we have seven Es, seven Ss, seven Ts and seven Js; this gives us three Is, three Ns, three Fs and three Ps. We can see that the I, N, F and P preferences are outnumbered in this organization, and the dominant group type is ESTJ. When we know this we are aware that the desires and behaviour of E, S, T and J win over I, N, F and P. We can then decide if ESTJ is the best group type for our organization, and if the work is largely dealing with production and distribution in a traditional way ESTJ is just what is needed.

But it may be that our organization spends much of its time adjusting to fluctuations in the market, and its sales, which involve all ten staff at times, are achieved mainly by persuasive personal communication. This is a situation that TJs are less at ease with, but in which FPs are likely to react well. In this situation knowing the group type is ESTJ helps this organization to see the need for more F and P. If they have the opportunity to recruit another member of staff they can ensure he or she is an FP type.

Only when we are aware of type can we see the need to balance this in an organization. With the ESTJ organization above it is more likely we would recruit someone who fitted in with the dominant group type. When we choose people to work with us we may think we choose people who are different from us, but most of us choose people who are similar, because we sense they are easy to get along with. And they are, but this may bring other problems, as we may all overlook vital work because no one is aware it needs doing.

Most businesses need different – even opposite – types to make them successful. It does make for more stress in working together, but a better balance of information is available to everyone, and a better balance of judgment. With different types around there are other advantages: small jobs which can be difficult and irritating for one type may be done with pleasure and ease by another.

Here is an example of this from a small manufacturing company:

An INTJ, working on future plans for the company, had his desk near the door where customers came in. He was given the job of welcoming them and finding out what they required. It was not long before he found this irksome, partly because his thoughts were far away in planning for the future of the business, and partly because it did not come easily to him to be warm and welcoming to customers and to find out what they wanted. Not far away an ESFJ was working at her desk, where she spent most of her day doing letters on the word processor; there were times when she would have liked to chat to someone – ESFJs are *very* sociable people. It was suggested to them that they might change work positions. This allowed the INTJ to work without interruption in order to concentrate on his planning. It brought the sociable ESFJ near the door to greet customers and find out their needs, something she loves. In fact very little change was made, and both continue to do their normal work, but both types are happier and able to work a little better.

Temperament and work satisfaction

As well as being aware of our different types at work we can become more conscious of our differences in temperament. Chapter 5 gives us a general idea of the Four Temperaments, and this section looks at how these are likely to affect us in the work we do. It is interesting for us to note the different attitudes of the temperaments to their work, and the different ways in which they set about this.

The type of work we do and how we set about this holds immense importance for us, as this can bring us deep personal satisfaction and fulfilment. It may seem strange to suggest that our work can hold meaning and significance for us. Yet it does. Only when the diverse needs of our temperament are met do we find this satisfaction and fulfilment. If we find this we produce our best and are happy, as we find meaning and significance through the work we do.

Here are some of the ways in which the four temperaments find satisfaction at work, and how they are likely to behave.

NF temperament (ENFJ, INFJ, ENFP and INFP)

NFs' attention is directed towards people. Even if they are working in a production industry they give their main energy to the people they work with. NFs are concerned for people's welfare, they are sensitive to their problems and are sympathetic and understanding.

They can work in many jobs provided they have opportunities for pleasing and helping people. Above all they like to appreciate people and bring about their emotional and personal growth. They have a unique insight and compassion into the feelings of others, and can use this in public relations, teaching or any work where it is important to communicate with people. NFs believe everyone shares their own lifelong search for identity.

NFs find it hard to face up to unpleasantness and they try to avoid this. Their desire to please may mean they take on too many commitments – especially if they are Ps – and they have a constant struggle to fulfil these on time; and in identifying with others' feelings they can get overloaded with others' problems and find this takes up much of their time and emotions. NFs need ongoing appreciation and affirmation of what they do at work, and without this they can sink into depression.

NFs like to bring their unique characteristics to any work they do. They need their work to be personal, and business is carried out at this level. When they speak to other people they do this in a persuasive manner. For NFs business is not merely the transaction of goods, but a way of promoting harmony between people. For this reason they often choose work which makes use of their counselling and facilitating skills, work in psychology or psychiatry or personnel. Working with language and literature also pleases them and they are outstanding teachers of these, able to pass on a deep and penetrating understanding to their pupils.

If we have NFs on our staff they bring a personal touch to their work, make the workplace more human and encourage staff to do their best.

NT temperament (ENTJ, INTJ, ENTP and INTP)

Work is highly important to NTs and their lives revolve around this. It is essential for them to have some project or idea in which their mind is engaged, and any work they do needs to have scope for future improvement. NTs are the designers of the future.

NTs can visualize projects and plans happening; they can see the working of these plans and how systems operate and connect. But if they need to explain these they may do so too succinctly, and others may not be given enough details. Therefore, they may not be good communicators or persuasive with their colleagues, and as they use words sparingly they are not usually socially inclined at work.

NTs value intelligence, and if they can make use of this at work they enjoy it. They are good at analysing plans, and business is usually approached in a scientific manner. Colleagues may see NTs as cold and non-conformist as it does not come easily to them to express warmth and appreciation.

It is hard for NTs to be patient with the day-to-day mundane details at work as their minds are always leaping ahead to the future. Their ability to think clearly ahead means they may be inclined to be impatient with those who cannot follow their reasoning.

NTs need to work where they can invent, design, plan and organize projects. Others may see them as restless and striving. Maintaining a business does not fulfil their desire for improvement, and they may start their own business in order to make use of their ability for invention.

Working out the theory of a plan and the ways in which it might happen occupies a lot of the NTs' time. Routine work with no creativity frustrates them. They are outstanding at dreaming up a project, and if they have the help of a more concrete person to see to the practical details this is likely to be highly successful.

If we have NTs on our staff they prevent stagnation at work. They can visualize how things will be in the future, and can make plans to put this into action.

SJ temperament (ESTJ, ISTJ, ESFJ and ISFJ)

We know how realistic, practical and well organized SJs are, and how concerned they are for safety and security. We can see they are keen to support established institutions and are good at looking after our money. We know we can expect them to be drawn to work that makes use of these qualities.

We find SJs in most businesses. They are the ones who keep our businesses going, being happy to see to the practical day-to-day details. They inspect what needs inspecting, supervise what needs supervising, and see that people and things are monitored and guarded. They look after the paperwork of a company, checking facts and figures carefully. They are generally successful in business as they are good at economics, and careful and responsible with goods and products. They expect to work hard and to be industrious. They tackle their work in a traditional manner and other types may consider them 'behind the times'.

People at work soon find out they can rely on SJs, and they appreciate this. We are likely to depend on them for their ability to see to practical details. Other temperaments may see SJs as conservative and set in their ways. They may feel SJs are rule-bound and unadaptable.

SJs do well in the business world as they have plenty of commonsense and a good understanding of how to run businesses successfully. They work well at looking after products, manage their time well and are responsible about providing a good service. They check goods, maintain them and store them carefully. If goods have to be moved or mailed this is all under control and the details are seen to reliably. Places of work are looked after with care. SJs may go into medicine and hospital work as well as working in banks, accounting, insurance and teaching.

If we have SJs on our staff they bring decisiveness and orderly methods to any work they do. They can always be relied upon to carry out their responsibilities.

SP temperament (ESTP, ISTP, ESFP and ISFP)

We find SPs in a variety of businesses, but their qualities at work are rarely understood. We see their concrete realism, their awareness of what is happening around them and their ability to turn disasters to advantage. Yet few of us appreciate their unique way of bargaining and negotiating. They love doing this, and have a highly developed sense of what is happening at the moment; they are not bothered with regulations, principles or matters which other temperaments may feel relate to the situation. So they are free to move things around and negotiate anything, and they usually do.

Making a deliberate choice of career may be difficult for SPs as they function best when they are free to go with the flow of life, changing what they do as the circumstances demand. If there is a situation or set-up in trouble they come in and do what is best to improve or rectify this. SPs are also good at setting up a business and getting it going. Once the business is going they lose interest in maintaining it, and it often fails due to inattention to regular details.

At heart SPs are craftspeople and workmen; they have a feel for working with tools and materials. Many are artistically gifted, and learn their craft with unusual speed and ease. If this is not their business they are likely to be involved with art or craft in their leisure time.

SPs need to be doing something active – paperwork and future theories do not hold their interest. They do not waste their energy on fruitless tasks. They need work which provides an element of competition, adventure and excitement, as they get bored easily. Commitments made yesterday may be forgotten today unless someone reminds them. They enjoy travel, finding this less tiring than other people. At work they need to use their five senses.

SPs are happy when they can act on the world around them. They enjoy work which allows them to be dramatic and entertaining. The Es are convincing in what they say, and they promote themselves and their businesses well; Is may have more difficulty doing this. Work related to machines, vehicles and tools makes use of their concrete, mechanical knowledge. The social side of work gives them immense enjoyment as they are well up with the latest in food, fashion and entertainment. They may do well in the musical or artistic world.

If we have SPs on our staff they cope well with the unexpected at work and are good at getting things to happen. They are adaptable to changes at work.

We can see how some of these differences work out in action by looking at examples of how the four temperaments react in similar situations.

Not long ago the general manager of a motor parts distribution company called an unexpected meeting of his four managers on a Monday morning. This was to let them know that the company was closing down one of the distribution centres. The NF manager became emotional, wanting to know what was being done to look after the welfare of the staff. The NT did not say much, and took the news coolly, appearing uninvolved; what he did say was that the closure would make a big difference to the future plans of the company. The SJ was anxious, saying he thought the changes would be upsetting to everyone in the company, and he came out with a number of points which he felt could go wrong with the closure. And the SP immediately got charged up and excited, and wanted to dash off to the centre and see if he could find a way around the problem.

With these different reactions to the same piece of news it was no wonder there was some difficulty in reaching agreement as to how best to manage the closure. Yet the four reactions gave the general manager a much wider perspective on the problem than he would have had by consulting with only one or two temperaments. If he had given weight to the opinions of all four temperaments he would have seen the importance of the different aspects of the problem. These included:

– looking after the welfare of the staff involved in the closure
– paying attention to the difference the closure would make to the future of the company
– looking into the problems arising from the closure which the SJ was aware of
– letting the SP come up with practical suggestions which might avoid the closure anyway.

Whatever decisions were finally taken it would have been beneficial to consider all of these points.

Here is another example of the differing views of the four temperaments at work, and how these were put into action to everyone's advantage.

A factory was planning to refurbish its out-of-date staff canteen. The project manager, an INTJ, called a meeting of the four staff representatives on the committee. He took care to let people see the plans in advance, and during the meeting he gave a further explanation of these to everyone. Without rushing people he allowed time for all of them to speak.

The NF representative felt the most important thing was to

provide surroundings where staff could pass a happy lunch hour. She was not particularly interested in the practicalities of the project. Her ideas would include decorating the room in a restful way, but the main thing was to provide an atmosphere where staff could engage in personal conversation. Small tables would be better than large ones for this, and the purpose of the lunch break was to help everyone to feel restored during lunch, so they could return to work emotionally strengthened for the afternoon.

The NT could not enthuse over these ideas; indeed he felt a bit scornful of them as they took no account of problems which might arise in the future. The SJ, though not against the ideas, could not enthuse either as she felt they were not primarily practical. And the SP felt it was more important to provide for the staff to have a good time than to provide for them to have personal interaction.

The NT representative felt the most important thing was to plan the present design with an eye to the future. He criticized some of the proposed plans, and put forward some ideas of his own that made good sense. His ideas allowed for the canteen to be enlarged and more staff to be catered for if the factory were to expand.

The NF could see the value of taking the future into account, provided that the personal lives of the staff were put first. The SJ could not get herself interested in planning the future of something that was not yet realized in the present! And the SP wanted to make the new canteen as exciting as possible now rather than look to the future.

The SJ representative felt distressed by the whole idea of refurbishing the canteen. She agreed the canteen was old fashioned, but felt it still functioned well in practice and it gave the staff a sense of solidity and security. She felt the disruption caused by the actual process of refurbishment would upset the routine of the staff, and a modern canteen would be unlikely to provide a solid and secure atmosphere. She suggested they might have a subcommittee to consider if it was possible to make some improvements to the canteen without having to go for total refurbishment.

The NF wanted to improve the canteen for the sake of making the staff happy, and was therefore not inclined to be enthusiastic about the SJ's desires to keep it as it was. The NT was all for changing things, and not at all keen to listen to the SJ praising the canteen's present values. And the SP, who saw the opportunity for making the lunch hour more fun and active, was keen to get away from the old-fashioned canteen.

The SP representative felt the new canteen should be made more exciting. He felt it should provide space for staff to be able to enjoy themselves and have a good time during their lunch hour; he suggested a bar with a seated area, together with some simple sports facilities like table tennis and snooker. If all of these were within the same area as the dining tables people could move around and do things as well as have their lunch.

The NF was against this, feeling that too much activity could prevent staff being more personal and getting together more intimately. The NT felt the SP's ideas would make it difficult to alter the canteen in the future. And the SJ dreaded the thought of a canteen which might lack organization and become a place with little discipline.

As we have seen the project manager was an INTJ, and therefore an NT temperament. He found, as we would expect, that he favoured the NT representative's view. But, with his knowledge of temperament, he made sure he gave weight to the other views as well. The end result took into account:

– the NF's desire to provide an atmosphere where staff could relax and relate personally to one another. This was provided at one end of the area
– the NT's desire to adjust the designs to provide a solution for the present, which also allowed room for improvement and expansion for the future
– the SJ's desire for giving further consideration to the project before taking a final decision. After doing this she saw the need for the new canteen, and gave her support to making the practical disruption as smooth as possible
– the SP's desire for fun and activity by providing an attractive bar area with indoor games nearby.

In the end everyone felt they got what they wanted. It was surprising how this helped them to feel enthusiastic about supporting the project as a whole, even to wanting everyone else's part to work out well.

This chapter gives us an idea of some of the ways in which we can avoid conflict and improve our situation at work, and we have seen the importance of giving consideration to our temperament. There are many more situations at work which can be improved as our understanding of type and temperament grows.

8

Education: What Happens
in the Classroom

From the moment we are born – and probably before this – we start taking in information about the world around us and begin to learn new things.

All of us learn in different ways. We can see children enjoying different things at an early age: they have favourite toys, are drawn to different people and play different games. It is not long before children in the same family can be seen to be unique individuals. These differences show up clearly in the way in which children learn about the world.

In our early years at school we have less choice over what we do, but as we move on to secondary school our natural tendencies become apparent and we are able to affect our individuality through choices.

To a large extent, the way in which we absorb information and learn depends on our type; similarly, in order to glean the most from information available, it has to be accessible to our type.

How we take in information

When Es learn about things they usually speak about them, which helps them confirm what they understand. Children generally tell everyone what they know, so it is easy for others to see this. With Is this is less apparent as they continue to assimilate information internally before they are likely to talk about it. Children, too, may keep their knowledge inside themselves. If we judge people by their outward behaviour it would appear that Es are quicker and brighter, but this is not the case.

We already know that Ss and Ns take in information in different ways, the Ss taking in the facts and what is actually there, and the Ns taking in things in ways that link them by pattern and relationship to other knowledge. INtuitives need to know the theory of something before they understand how they can use it. Whether we are S or N must be the greatest difference in our way of absorbing and dealing with information.

Thinkers like information presented to them logically and reasonably, especially the NTs. They are less inclined to learn material that is presented to them subjectively. As children, they need to be given a good reason to do something before they are willing to co-operate. Feelers, whether adults or children, are more likely to do their work to please their teacher, and to help out in class without needing reasons, and they can be put off learning if there is disharmony in the class.

Judgers feel more confident when the teacher tells them what material they will cover, and then sticks to this. They like to know what to expect, and P teachers who chop and change things throw Js off balance. Perceivers prefer not to know what is coming, taking the information as it comes. If they are told in detail about a lesson or course this spoils it for them, and they may lose interest even before the lesson starts. Most Ps need help in organizing their material for projects and written work.

How we learn: consider temperament

One of the ways in which we get a good idea of how children learn is by looking at the four temperaments. Of course school is only part of our learning process, and these descriptions relate to the whole of a child's world as they learn. They help us to see that all of us have different kinds of intelligence and that we excel at different kinds of things.

INtuitive–Feeling (NF) temperament

NF children are invariably popular with teachers, as they are inspiring to teach. They like to please others, both teachers and their fellow pupils. They feel responsible for the atmosphere in the classroom at an early age, and try to look after others and be sensitive to their feelings. Their relationships are highly important to them, as is understanding themselves and those around them. NF children are emotional and idealistic, and often experience big disappointments by having too high expectations.

NFs enjoy learning and see knowledge as having meaning and significance, everything relating to everything else. If they have teachers who give them little personal attention they find it hard to learn. They put themselves out to please everyone and need encouragement from teachers as they go along. They like class discussions where everyone contributes, and dislike arguments and conflict.

They are quick to pick up on learning their alphabet and learning to read. Language comes easily to NF children and often they can express themselves in words beyond their years. They become avid readers, learning much from books. As they get older they enjoy literature, which they read subjectively, reacting with sensitivity to stories. It is harder for them to see things objectively.

INtuitive–Thinking (NT) temperament

NT children have a thirst for knowledge from an early age. They value intelligence even when young, and only respect their teacher if they feel he or she is competent to speak on their subject. If they are interested in something NT children go off and find out more about this on their own, often acquiring a mass of knowledge about a subject that interests them. They take in information in abstract ways and enjoy brainstorming sessions. Often they are bright academically.

When they learn things they like the information to be backed up by logic and reason. NT children are little scientists, and often end up in work that needs research and has a scientific basis. In class, they can be difficult for teachers to deal with as they may not be the most co-operative members, sometimes appearing socially inept and ungraceful.

If NT children are presented with isolated facts they find this unsatisfactory, as they need to understand what is behind the facts and what the facts relate to. Some children may appear odd, especially the INTs, as they may not join in with other children's games and general talk. They are independent children, going their own way rather than the way of the family or their school. Arranging and ordering things systematically comes easily to the NT child, who is also ingenious and enjoys working out logical ideas.

Sensing–Judging (SJ) temperament

SJ children need to do things and to handle things rather than store up theory in their minds. They take information in through their five senses. They learn by absorbing things step-by-step, in linear fashion, and by having a secure environment in which to work. They are unlikely to go off and make their own discoveries. They answer factual questions quickly as they have good memories for facts. Work of a practical nature suits SJs best, and they like to work towards a goal or end product. SJ children like to be told what to do and how they should do it, and they need their lessons presented in an orderly manner. They do not like undirected work or projects, as they have difficulty with more creative and inventive work.

Teachers can depend on SJ children, and they carry out their work responsibly. The SJ child fits in easily at school from an early age. They have a sense of belonging to their class and enjoy the structure and routine of school. Jobs like class monitor or other practical responsibilities given to the SJ will be done regularly and thoroughly. Even young SJs can be seen trying to be well behaved and giving service, and getting a good report is important to them.

Sensing–Perceiving (SP) temperament

SP children are similar to SJ children in their need to learn by *doing* things; they seldom learn much by writing or saying things. In school they need to be allowed some mobility and freedom of action. They learn from pictures and films, and enjoy drawing. If they can make something which relates to the subject this helps them to learn about it. They find out by asking people questions.

If they can play games they enjoy these. They need to be involved in doing something during a lesson; theory and lectures are too abstract for them. Visual things attract SPs, and they like fun and entertainment. Their senses of sight, sound, smell, taste and feel need to be used, and they learn spontaneously from what is around. Like SJs, SPs learn through their five senses, and are best when they are given practical assessments. Competitions, risk and excitement stimulate them.

Their early years in school are likely to provide them with what they need. As they get older lessons tend to become too theoretical for them. When this happens they lose interest in their work and may become disruptive and develop behaviour problems. Often, the teachers – who are more likely to be SJ or NF in primary school – may feel SPs are backward or dull. But when the SP is allowed to be active and move around as they learn they are likely to do well. If not – and they are required to sit still and keep information in their minds only – SPs may well fall behind in class and never move on to higher education. There are few SPs who last long in higher education as this is rarely geared to their needs. An SP child needs to see that their lessons are not just theoretical but can be put to some practical and active use in the world.

Teachers

This has given us some idea of the different needs of children as they learn about the world, and we can see these learning characteristics at an early age. Depending on our circumstances as we grow older, we develop these characteristics to a greater or lesser degree. When we leave school we may become students, and whatever we do we go on learning all our lives. We learn in our own way, and when we choose work we instinctively opt for something which interests us and appeals to our way of learning.

As we become adults some of us become teachers, and we teach in our own style. A teacher at primary level, who is one type and temperament, has up to sixteen different types in his/her class. The children who are the same or a similar type to the teacher feel at home with him/her. These children will receive information in a way they enjoy, and they will find it easy to talk to their teacher; equally, it is likely that the teacher finds them easy-to-manage members of the class.

But the children who are dissimilar to their teacher are likely to have the most difficulty, and the teacher is likely to find them the most difficult to teach. It is the same with adults, and we find it easiest to learn with someone who is like us. The slight exception to this is the NF teacher, who has the ability to see how others see, and then sees how to teach them.

We can understand different teachers' attitudes and methods better by looking at temperament.

INtuitive–Feeling (NF) teachers

NFs are usually regarded as being inspiring teachers, and a comparatively large number of them choose this profession as it makes use of their gifts. They believe that teaching is about the unfolding of personalities, and they like to be part of the facilitation process. Most children are drawn to them as they have a personal and caring manner.

NF teachers are often found teaching arts subjects such as languages, literature and music. They have a natural profound understanding of these and can communicate them with ease, making their pupils enthusiastic.

NFs encourage pupil interaction through personal relationships, and they themselves relate personally to their pupils, bringing a warm and accepting atmosphere into the classroom. NF teachers like to involve their class in lessons. They initiate class discussions, encouraging everyone to take part, and they set up small group projects.

The commitment and involvement of the teachers places some strain on them personally and they frequently become overloaded both physically and emotionally. Sometimes they take on the troubles of their pupils, feeling involved in these. NF teachers believe education is to encourage personal development in children.

INtuitive–Thinking (NT) teachers

NT teachers are drawn to higher education and we see more of them in universities and colleges than we do in primary schools. Not too many of them go in for teaching and some of them drop out when they find they are unhappy in the system. As they value intelligence – as they understand this – and science they are likely to teach the more scientific subjects, as well as maths and more abstract subjects like languages and philosophy. One of the reasons we lack science teachers is the small number of NTs.

NTs dislike using more words than they have to, and teachers try to communicate to children and students without unnecessary explanations. This works well with the NT children, but the others often feel the teachers are going too fast without enough details. They may push the class along without finding out whether the class is ready for this.

NT teachers have high standards for themselves and expect high standards from their classes, but they are unlikely to be lavish in their encouragement and praise. They use lectures, tests and projects to teach, and their own love of learning is usually communicated to their classes. They are better with bright students, as they have little patience with students who are slow. NT teachers encourage children to increase their knowledge and intelligence.

Sensing–Judging (SJ) teachers

SJ teachers are the backbone of the teaching profession, bringing social and community responsibility into schools. They have a strong sense of history and tradition, and they enjoy contributing to carrying this on. They fit in easily with the teaching system, supporting and enforcing rules and regulations.

SJs tend to teach more practical and factual subjects like history, geography and home economics. They are good at teaching business and commercial practices. SJ teachers like to prepare children to live in the practical world and to be dependable citizens. They are likely to encourage children to take up steady jobs like accountancy, banking, insurance and teaching.

Their method of teaching is step-by-step in a well planned and organized way. They check that children are learning by tests and repetition. With plenty of SJ teachers the SJ children feel at home in the atmosphere and environment at school. SJ teachers are patient with those who make an effort, and children get a sense of stability from them. They encourage children to become useful and reliable.

Sensing–Perceiving (SP) teachers

Our present teaching system draws very few SP teachers, with the result that SPs are under-represented in the profession. SP teachers, as we might expect, need an environment which allows them to be active and spontaneous in their work. Few of them are drawn to teaching, which is built on a structured timetable and well planned lessons.

But SPs make exciting teachers, bringing activity and entertainment into their classes. They usually teach in active subjects like art, music, drama and sport. They are less likely to have degrees in more abstract subjects. They like to do things with children: they will demonstrate things and show pictures and films; they may bring in games and competitions. The prescribed syllabus may be ignored in the excitement of getting involved with something else that catches their attention. Homework may not be set, or may not even be marked.

SPs frequently do not last in teaching as they become frustrated with the rules and the system, and find there is little room for them to be themselves. This is unfortunate, as there are many SP children who need role models in childhood. We have already seen that SP children often do not fit into school, and one of the reasons is that we have so few SP teachers. With more SP teachers the SP children would enjoy school better and be inclined to learn more. SP teachers encourage children to live spontaneously, finding things out for themselves.

If we look at children we can see their different learning patterns in their types and temperaments, and we can see the same learning patterns in adults. If we look at the ways in which the temperaments learn as adults we can confirm this.

Learning in adults: consider temperament

INtuitive–Feeling (NF) temperament

NFs learn from life experiences, and for them personal growth plays a large part in their learning process. They experience the world globally, relating each and every happening to the wider world.

Learning needs to relate personally to NFs, making a difference to people's lives. Like the NTs, NFs take in information in more abstract ways, fitting this in to their view of life in general. Like the NTs, too, they are more academic than the SJs and SPs.

NFs bring a commitment to learning provided there is personal involvement for them and others. They often bring unique insight to their studies. They need to be recognized as individuals, and they need to be valued for what they contribute personally.

INtuitive–Thinking (NT) temperament

Learning is a life-long process for the NT, but they need to feel their teacher is intelligent before they accept what is being taught. Above all NTs enjoy learning by themselves, and if they are interested in a subject they study on their own. They need to feel their study is leading somewhere.

NTs take in information in abstract ways, analysing and sorting this into related compartments. They are prepared to find out what they want by research, and the information they gather is projected into the future. If data appears illogical or productivity is inefficient NTs are scornful, as they value efficiency.

They often push themselves unnecessarily as they have high standards. They need to be valued for their logical minds and forward thinking.

Sensing–Judging (SJ) temperament

As they get to the end of school SJs usually have a good idea of the work they are aiming towards. With their abilities they can go into most forms of business and commerce, and all the traditional professions such as banking, accountancy, insurance and medicine.

Like the SPs, they continue to learn as they do things. But unlike the SPs they learn in an orderly manner, acquiring facts and practical knowledge bit by bit. Isolated facts are tucked away inside them, ready to use if they are needed.

SJs learn what is needed in the world and their community, and they try to contribute something practical. They need to be valued for being responsible and hard working.

Sensing–Perceiving (SP) temperament

School holds less and less appeal for SPs as they get older. As lessons contain more lectures and abstractions the SP gets very bored.

SPs learn well from short visual presentations, especially if they can then do something related to this. If they can make or construct something, or involve drama or sport, their attention is held.

Often, most of their learning is acquired through practical experience after leaving school. These abilities are developed through touching things and using their eyes, ears, noses and mouths. SPs learn from knowing what is going on around them, and they need to be valued for living as the ultimate realists.

We can remind ourselves that learning in school begins as a more S activity and becomes more N as education progresses. With a large number of SJ teachers, especially at primary level, schools tend to be run on SJ lines. In secondary education this is balanced by the NF teachers, who have a strong influence in facilitating the personal development of pupils. The number of N pupils increases as higher education becomes more theoretical and academic, particularly at university, and the number of N teachers increases in secondary and higher education too.

It is significant that exams and tests are usually set by N teachers, and these exams obviously suit Ns more than Ss. N ideas of knowledge and intelligence is not the same as S ideas of these.

9

Families

Recent years have made us more aware of the personal needs of the individual. We find it easier to accept different ways of living and being, and we have become more tolerant of one another. But as our personal needs become more accepted, so the family comes under pressure. Many changes are taking place in family life, and there can be few of us who do not feel involved. The cohesive family unit of father, mother and children is becoming even more elusive, and most of us are now part of some form of extended family. It is easy to see the pressures this can cause.

All families benefit from some awareness of type differences as the individual members of any family are likely to have different needs, values, hopes and ambitions. Perhaps it is surprising that families manage to live together at all. But before we go on to look at how these differences affect us we can take note of two points.

Family dynamics

First, our view of the world around us comes from our experiences within our family. It is easy for us to feel that all families are like ours. They are not, of course, and we eventually discover this, and we have to adapt ourselves to a world outside where people differ from those in our family. Yet the influence of our parents and family lay foundations in us from our earliest years when we are at our most receptive.

Second, our family relationships generate very strong feelings within us. We are placed with those who may or may not be like us, and somehow we have to get on together.

Influence or type

Let's consider some of the situations that are part of family life. Father is one type, and Mother is likely to be another. Their similarity – or lack of it – has a major effect on their children. If they are similar in type they are likely to agree about many things, and likely to enforce their own characteristics on their children. If, however, they are unlike in type their children may be pulled in different directions, but they are exposed to a wider experience of the world.

Other influences become apparent. The dominant parent is likely to urge his or her characteristics on the children more forcefully, especially if he or she spends more time with them than the other. And any preference that is shared by a child is usually spotted and capitalized on, often for the benefit of the child but sometimes to the detriment of its opposite preference.

If we look from a child's viewpoint we can see that a child of similar type to a parent finds an ally in him/her, and is likely to prefer this parent. Whereas a child of a markedly different type is likely to have disagreements with this parent. The same is true for brothers and sisters. Similar types have much in common and usually enjoy being together; opposite types are frequently at variance. Yet it can take only one different preference to cause dissension and disharmony.

We can see that within the family set-up some preferences may dominate. Here are the types of one family:

Father   ISTJ
Mother   ENTJ
Daughter ESFJ
Son   ESTP

In this family three are Es, three are Ss, three are Ts and three are Js. There is only one I, one N, one F and one P. It is clear that the E,S,T and J preferences 'win' over the I,N,F and P preferences. We can say that ESTJ dominates this family, and they are likely to come across to others as an ESTJ family.

We can look further to see how these preferences might work out within this family. Three of them are Es, only Father is an I. The three Es are bound to talk a lot between themselves, all of them wondering why Father does not join in. Father needs to withdraw to get his personal space, and as he does this the other three pressurize him into being more sociable; this causes him to withdraw even further.

Three of them are Ss; Mother is the only N. The conversation of three Ss is likely to be about the events and practical details of the world around them, and the day-to-day happenings of their lives. Mother is alone in her more abstract thinking and if she verbalizes her ideas to the rest of the family they are unable to follow her. Mother feels frustrated and the three Ss often feel she is 'in the clouds'.

It is the same with T and F as three of this family are Ts, only the ESFJ daughter is F. She has trouble making them understand her concern with her own and other people's feelings. The three Ts approach things more impersonally and rationally, making it hard for the F daughter to explain how she feels about matters. This family is dominant in T and the one F considers her values and feelings are given little attention.

Apart from the son, who is ESTP, the rest of this family are Js. The

Js are well-organized, plan ahead and do things on time. The P son constantly annoys them as he refuses to be pinned down by arranging things in advance, and he decides what he does as he goes along. If they go out as a family he is rarely ready on time, infuriating the three Js, who gather together and turn on him. This family is J dominant and the P feels the family are trying to control him.

Later in this chapter we look at ways in which some of these family conflicts might be resolved.

When we have dominant preferences in a family these become the expected way for the family members to behave. When the children are young these dominant preferences come from the parents, and as the children grow up their own preferences fight for acknowledgment. At school parents encourage their own preferences, and when the children choose a career they may be steered towards work which reflects the parents' choice rather than the natural preferences of the child.

We can look at some of the things different parents feel are important. These are the qualities they encourage and urge their children to develop.

Parents' influence

Extraverts urge their children to be outgoing and sociable. When they see them being more withdrawn and playing on their own they encourage them to join other children and groups. Extraverts have a fear that their children will be withdrawn, and they make every effort to see that they join in activities and make friends.

Introvert parents find E children demanding, and urge them to engage in quieter activities, hoping they will come to value things they can do on their own. Introverts enjoy doing something quiet with their children, but generally do not put too much pressure on their children to be I. Possibly because they are not noisy themselves, the I parent can take pleasure in observing their E child being boisterous and outgoing.

Sensers spend a lot of time telling their children facts, they feel it is important to give them factual knowledge of the world to teach them how to cope in it. They are often painstaking about teaching them practical tasks. These can range from tying their shoelaces to getting a mortgage.

INtuitives are less likely to spend too much time telling their children facts, and more likely to offer them ideas and possibilities to open up their minds. They are more concerned with how their children can talk *about* things than what they can do in practical terms.

Thinkers urge their children to develop logical minds. If this does not come naturally to the child, Ts point out their illogical reasoning to them. They teach them to work things through so that their arguments make sense. Thinkers may not have much patience with a child who comes up with a woolly or emotional response.

Feelers urge their children to develop understanding and caring for those around them. Feelers demonstrate this in their own lives, and take pains to see that their children show consideration and appreciation towards others. To F parents this is more important than logic or firmness.

Judgers urge a well-organized life on their children. When their children are young Js organize their lives for them, but as they grow older they are expected to do this for themselves. Children who are late or unprepared for school or family events are sure to annoy J parents, who expect them to be productive, decisive and have things ready on time.

Perceivers are more easy-going as parents, tending to let their children find out about life for themselves. They are less strict and more relaxed about time. P parents like to give their children many opportunities to learn and experience a variety of things.

Parenting: consider temperament

If we are parents our temperament urges us to encourage our children to develop the characteristics we feel to be important. Here are some of the ways in which the four temperaments act as parents, and some of the things they try and teach their children.

NFs want to help their children become unique human beings who can bring insight and imagination to other people's lives. They take opportunities to expose them to a variety of creative opportunities, and to open their minds to different ways of thinking and feeling. It is hard for the NF parent to understand a child who has little imagination and is not interested in ideas, or one who is insensitive towards those around them.

NTs have high standards for their children and like them to develop their minds intellectually. They expect them to know their own minds and to talk logically about things. Their children are expected to expand their knowledge by using their thinking processes, and they have little patience with incompetence. It is hard for the NT to understand a child who lacks imagination and is unable to reason things.

SJs are concerned to train their children to become dependable and stable adults. They teach them to be responsible citizens, working to meet the needs of society. They urge them to work hard at school and to become sensible members of the family. It is hard for the SJ parent to understand a child who lives in a world of dreams and imagination; and the SJ parent has difficulty with a wayward child or one who seems unaware of time.

SPs are generally easy-going as parents, letting their children 'grow like weeds'. They teach them to be aware of the practicalities of what is happening around them, and to remember things. They point out realistic opportunities, and encourage their children to make the most of these. Like the SJ it is hard for the SP parent to understand a child who goes into a world of dreams and imagination, or one who does not notice what is going on in the world around them.

Children: type, temperament and behaviour

We have seen some of the things that parents of different types and temperaments urge upon their children. Now we can look at how children of different types and temperaments are likely to behave, and how they may respond in their families. Although we cannot ask children what type they are in their early years, it is often possible for us to see this at a young age.

Extraverts

Extravert children need other members of their family to acknowledge them, such as when they come into the house or even when they enter a room. Introvert parents seldom do this. Extravert children need parents and siblings to talk to them constantly, to comment on what they are doing or thinking. Without this Es pursue the Is in their family to get them to say something, and the Is hate this. Extraverts are generally quick to respond to suggestions, and swift to act. Because E children are more outgoing and tell us what they feel it is easier to understand them, and they tend to get positive feedback from those around them.

Introverts

Introvert children escape into their rooms frequently, spending a lot of time there. This is when the Es chase after them, disturbing their peace. Introverts may disappear for hours on solitary activities as they need to learn and absorb things at their own pace. They tend to be reticent, shy and quiet. Family friends and visitors seldom see the best of I children. A boisterous, noisy family is overpowering for an I child, who needs personal space to retreat to. Introvert children are usually more difficult to understand as they show us less of themselves.

Sensers

Sensing children like to be doing something, they enjoy being active and making things. They are generally quick to pick up on the necessary practical everyday tasks. They tend to live in the present, observing things around them, many of them noticing details at an early age. Factual stories of events that actually happened are remembered by them. If they have other S family members, which is likely, they repeat their news and their doings to each other. When they ask questions they like factual answers, and may get impatient if Ns reply in less definite terms. The great majority of children are Ss.

INtuitives

INtuitive children are less concrete, they often daydream and may not be fully in the present. Their toys and rooms may be arranged in a way that appears to be nonsensical; but to the N child there is some method and order, and all their objects have some relationship to one another. They enjoy more fictional stories which allow them to use their imagination, and they get upset if Ss in their family make fun of their creative ideas. There are far fewer N children, and S parents may feel they are odd or different.

Thinkers

Thinking children seldom respond to family rules unless they are given reasons for these, but if rules or requests make sense to them they fall in with them. Often they stand apart from family wrangles and do not get emotionally involved with these. If they do, they give their viewpoint in no uncertain terms. Natural family chat may not come easily to them. Even ET children may not show their affection or feelings outwardly, but their feelings are there inside them. Unless the F point of view is put to them logically they may be scornful of this.

Feelers

Feeling children like to please other members of the family, and may go out of their way to do this, as it is important for them to receive appreciation from others. They are generally quick to notice other people's feelings and reactions. Family wrangles are times when the F child, even if young, feels involved and may try and act as a mediator. Conflict and arguments in the family upset F children and they show their emotions readily to others. The Es especially can talk easily and are affectionate. Thinkers can upset them by their apparently cold attitude to life.

We can remind ourselves of the T/F bias here. As with everywhere else T girls and F boys may be regarded as not behaving 'normally'.

Judgers

Judging children depend on routine, and when this is changed can be upset, it takes away their structure. They like to be told about changes in advance, not have them suddenly sprung on them. J children are generally on time for school, for outings and other appointments. If they are given a job in the family they can be depended upon to do this at the right time. And if other family members do not do their share the J child may try to organize them. If P members of the family are unorganized or late for things this can annoy them immensely.

Perceivers

Perceiving children like to be given the freedom to find things out for themselves, they enjoy 'discovering' information and possibilities. They like surprises and are always looking for something new. They feel tied down if the family lives a life governed by strict routine as they have little need for order. P children are usually untidy. They can be unaware of time, especially the Ns, and they need reminding about most things.

Temperament, too, in children becomes apparent, and we can see this in different ways.

INtuitive–Feeling (NF) temperament

NF children need their family and those around them to be in harmony. They relate easily to others and are usually quite charming. Reading and language come easily to them, and they become avid readers; they like hearing imaginative stories and, being imaginative themselves, they create their own stories.

They like to discuss things with others, and like family members to share their thoughts and feelings. Conflict and criticism upset them immensely, and they flourish when given personal attention.

INtuitive–Thinking (NT) temperament

NT children may be precocious, asking many questions beyond their years. Asking questions and reading is their way of finding things out, and their knowledge is in their heads rather than in what they do. They may not fit in easily to the social side of family life, and may lack the charm of other temperaments.

They tend to be independent and nonconformist. Early on they develop their critical faculties, and use these to concentrate on things they consider worthwhile, being scornful of things they consider worthless.

100

Sensing–Judging (SJ) temperament

SJ children need a hierarchy, they like to know their place in the family. They see themselves as part of a larger family, and relate to each member, being conscious of the different levels and rights of each one. Since they depend on their place in the family they need a secure family, and family breakdown and change upset them immensely.

SJ children have little difficulty fitting in with family and school routine. If they are given small jobs either at home or school they carry these out reliably. They need to be praised for doing these.

Sensing–Perceiving (SP) temperament

Unlike the SJ children, SPs dislike hierarchy and fight against this. They need to be free to find out about life for themselves. As they are observant they find out by going off and *doing* things: they feel things, see things, smell things, touch things and taste things, and often they get messy doing this.

SP children like to be active, and they need excitement and variety. They are unlikely to spend hours reading a book. If they are allowed to be active and to do things, they are usually happy. They may enjoy playing a musical instrument, making something or playing an energetic game. Generally, they are good-natured.

Resolving conflicts

We can look back now to our family on p. 95, and see how some of the conflicts might be resolved. To do this each member needs to have some basic knowledge of type – understanding the needs of their own preferences and also *the needs of their opposite preferences*. Given this there is a strong probability that some of their conflicts will diminish. We can remind ourselves of their types: Father is ISTJ; Mother is ENTJ; Daughter is ESFJ; Son is ESTP. The first conflict is over E and I. With three Es in the family and only one I we see that E is dominant, and there is pressure on the father to be more E. The father feels he needs his peace and quiet, but feels guilty taking this. When everyone is aware of the needs of Es and Is, father does not have to feel guilty when he wants to be on his own, and the three Es can see why he needs this. In turn, Father sees that the rest of the family need interaction with one another, and lets them get on with this. The Es make some effort to tone down their boisterousness when Father is around. Father makes some effort to live out of his E when the family is all together, knowing he can return to his I without them resenting this.

When we look at S and N conflict in this family we see there are three Ss and only one N. Sensing is dominant, and the three Ss' conversation concerns their day-to-day doings. Ideas and concepts are not part of their communication with one another. As well as this the three Ss are all practical and capable in the home. Mother, the one N, feels she has no one with whom to share her thoughts. She is also aware that she is less capable at managing her share of the household tasks. When they become aware of S and N type differences, they all agree to listen to some of Mother's ideas without dismissing them, and Mother decides to value and make use of the family's S strengths by asking their advice and help over practical tasks in the home.

Since there are three Ts in this family, they are T dominant, and the F daughter struggles for recognition of her personal values. Every time the family discusses a topic she is shouted down by the Ts, who all consider her arguments woolly and illogical. Now they all have some understanding of T and F, the three Ts agree to listen to what she is saying, and to give some value to her way of making decisions. In turn, she agrees to try and see situations from a more logical viewpoint.

Finally, with J and P it is the son who is alone here. The three others like to plan their lives, making arrangements in advance and agreeing definite times to do things. None of them likes to change his/her arrangements once they have made them. The son feels all the others expect him to be tied down to family commitments, whereas he prefers to decide whether he joins in with these nearer the time. He also likes to go off when he feels like it to meet his friends or play sport. The family agrees to be less rigid about their arrangements, and not to mind if he does not join in. Equally, he agrees to commit himself to certain things that are part of the family routine.

This family makes use of other aspects of the different types and temperaments. Both Father and Mother are TJs – a combination of preferences that makes parents more inclined to be rigid and strict. Now they realize this they try to be a little more easy-going with the children. Father and daughter are SJ temperament. They share a need for a more traditional life and values. Mother is an NT, and she needs areas where she can think up new ideas, and being a J she also wants to put them into action. The SP son needs some freedom from restrictions. They are still an ESTJ-dominant family, but with an understanding of the different drives of their temperaments they are all more accepting of one another's needs.

How to get on with each other

Many families have become extended, making relationships more complex. Apart from grandparents or grandchildren there may be second wives or husbands plus their previous families. All these additions make more combinations of type. It is likely that any extended family unit comprises most of the preferences, and if we remind ourselves of some of the needs of each preference we can learn more about how these fit in with one another:

Es need to talk and have interaction with others.

Is need personal space and quiet.

Es can ensure they give Is their space by not expecting them to talk with them all the time.

Is can use their E side in order to communicate with Es, knowing they can return to their I when they want. (There is more about this in Chapter 12.)

Ss need to talk and act around practical, concrete things and their lives revolve around the details of these.

Ns' conversation often revolves around possibilities for the future, and they talk about things in less specific ways.

Ss can listen to Ns' ideas with more attention as Ns are good at thinking things up for the future.

Ns can learn from Ss about the concrete world as this is likely to benefit the home in practical ways.

Ts need discussions to be approached from a logical viewpoint.

Fs need discussions to include how the outcome affects people's lives.

Ts can listen and be willing to consider people's feelings more.

Fs can consider the logical viewpoint and try to look ahead to the consequences.

Js need to be able to plan and organize their lives at home.

Ps need freedom to be more spontaneous and flexible at home.

Js and Ps can agree on what they can organize together. The Ps should keep to their commitments; the Js can then organize themselves for other things.

As adults we may look back on our early years with happiness; we may look back with unhappiness. Most of us look back with a mixture of both. Whatever our family background, it provides us with our idea of the world and a way of understanding things. As we become mature adults we need to reassess ourselves in relation to our family, and also in relation to others. We need to look at other families, and we need to get to know other people well. This gives us a more rounded way of understanding the world.

But we need our childhood influences so that we have a yardstick by which to re-evaluate ourselves. We can then accept that our own family has given us many benefits and positive influences, and some of these are given by those whose types are different from ours. Without the experience of growing up in our family we might have been unaware of these differences, and this would have been to our detriment. We need to come to see that we have a unique contribution to bring to the world and a unique place to fill. In this way we grow from within our family' and develop into mature adults.

10

Attraction and Conflict
in Love

Since the world began men and women have been attracted to one another and have formed partnerships and marriages. Some of these have been on a temporary basis and others have been permanent. Until recently most marriages usually lasted until the death of one partner; but in recent years there have been changes in lifestyles. During the 1980s there was a massive increase in broken relationships – which nearly always causes considerable emotional anguish and misery as well as financial difficulties.

In spite of knowing that many relationships end disastrously, most couples get together with the fervent hope and intention that their relationship will last. Both partners are likely to feel they will stay together, and can see no reason for the liaison to flounder. Often a strong sense of agreement about lifestyles, shared interests and attitudes prevails. Sadly, though, this may be misleading.

After one week, one month, one year or even a half-century we may feel our relationship is utterly different from when it started. Qualities we found attractive in our partner may now irritate us; characteristics and behaviour that we take for granted in ourselves may not even be there in our partner. In short, we now see our partner as a very different person; different not only from ourself but from our initial perceptions. Reality can seem very harsh.

Yet our choice of partner has the greatest influence on determining our future life. The fusing of two separate, and possibly contrasting, lives produces a shared lifestyle, and creates the way in which the two will live together as a couple. However, the combination – or is it combustion? – of one type when joined with another type does have some predictable results. This chapter looks at some of the things that happen when the different types and temperaments link up as couples.

Similar or opposite?

Some of us choose a partner with either three or four preferences in common with ours, and with this we can expect a considerable amount of harmony. But even with one different preference we may experience conflict and misunderstanding. We can look, for example, at an ENFJ type. Living with an INFJ provides the greatest similarities, as they share temperament and an organized lifestyle. But the I's need for reflection and solitude is the opposite of the ENFJ's extremely talkative and outgoing manner. If the ENFJ has an ESFJ partner there is less in common, as the ESFJ's concrete and practical way of taking in information is contrary to the ENFJ's more impressionistic and general way, and this results in their decisions and actions being based on different information. If the ENFJ has an ENTJ partner there is more in common, sharing similar information gathering, and a difference only in how they arrive at decisions. And with the ENFP there is the shared NF temperament as with the INFJ, but here there is always conflict between the more organized lifestyle of the ENFJ and the more flexible one needed by the ENFP. And this is with only one different preference!

What if there are more? Two, three or even four different preferences? When we investigate our choice of partners we find some fascinating evidence is revealed – that we really *are* attracted to our opposites, and that we are likely to choose a partner who has at least two preferences different from ours, often more. Our understanding of type and temperament can help us to avoid some of these conflicts and to benefit from our differences. We can see that if half of our preferences are more developed it is natural for us to look for someone who provides the half of us which is less developed. The expression 'My other half' begins to make sense, and we can find the relationship balances us and makes us more complete.

If we are linked with a similar partner we can expect less conflict, but also less attraction. There may be no violent rows, but there may be no violent attraction either. Our strengths may be doubled but our weaknesses are likely to be doubled as well.

With a partner with two or more different preferences it is another story. There is more spark here, more tension, more attraction and the potential for a broader and fuller lifestyle. Each of us has something fresh to bring to the other, and as we are likely to have different interests it may be easier for us both to retain our individuality.

Opposites definitely attract, and it is easy to see why. A partner with different preferences provides us with the things we cannot give ourselves. There is also much more likelihood of conflict and disagreement.

What does each type want from his/her partner? Some of us may say we want specific qualities, but most of us are hard-pressed to articulate definite ideas about this. Perhaps it is the other way round? It is not that we want our partner to demonstrate specific qualities so much as we want him or her to allow *us* to live out the characteristics of our type.

Whether we are more likely to do this with someone who is similar or with someone who is different, we are unfortunately not able to predict.

We might also ask what is it that attracts us to one another? If we look at this in type terms it is not difficult to see where some of the attractions lie. The E is drawn to the depth and concentration of the I, fascinated to discover there is more to the I than we meet on the surface; the I is attracted to the vivacious and outgoing E, delighted to find someone who is at ease in the outside world. The realistic S is drawn to the ingenuity of the N, amazed at the N's insight and imagination; and the N is attracted to the down-to-earth and practical S, delighted to find someone who is grounded in the real world. The T is drawn to the humane and yielding F, appreciating their skill with people and their understanding manner; and the F is attracted to the firm and logical T, valuing the T's ability to be objective and cool-headed. And the controlled J is drawn to the easy-going P, delighted to find someone who brings excitement and spontaneity to life; and the P is attracted to the well-organized J, knowing the J brings structure and control to life.

We may admire the qualities we lack, but unless we discover, understand and accept our differences we may not last together. All of us seem to be attracted to and admire the qualities we lack, but, the trouble is, *we want our partner to have these other qualities as well as our own*: we want our partner to be different and yet the same! None of us can be like this, and if someone is different from us they cannot be the same. We use the expression of two people being 'poles apart' and sometimes differences between people are so immense that it is unrealistic to expect them to live together. But most differences can be understood and appreciated, and then there is a chance for both to benefit.

If we look at the four pairs of preferences we can see some of the things that cause clashes and misunderstandings in our relationships. We also look at ways in which we can avoid these conflicts.

Extraversion and Introversion (E and I)

Extraverts are out and about in the outside world more than Is. Introverts are more likely to be at home, possibly reading, reflecting or, if IS, doing something quietly. Extraverts therefore are likely to have more experience of the outside world, and when they choose a partner may make a more informed choice. On the other hand, they may not have spent much time considering – being too busy to do this – and may make their decisions hastily. Introverts like to have time to consider, and think before committing themselves to anything.

Extraverts are also more likely to be the ones to make the initial choice, being more outgoing, more willing to make bridges to reach others and also coming to their decisions quicker. Introverts may find they have been chosen before they know what is happening! Male Is are often grabbed by female Es before the I has had time to consider if this is a relationship he really wants. By then it is too late as he is carried away by the E's enthusiasm and vivacity, and he is captured. IT males (there are more T males than T females) are often chosen by EF females – the females providing the outgoing warmth that the IT male may lack. Extraverts and introverts choose each other frequently; there is a definite attraction here. We see them around us all the time.

William and Jane, a busy couple with a young family, arranged a babysitter so they could have a meal out together and some uninterrupted time. William, an E, thought: 'We don't get out often, we'll have a proper chance to talk. I can tell Jane about my idea for the gift shop without the children always butting in.'

Jane, an I, thought: 'We don't get out often, we'll have a chance to be quiet together without the children interrupting.'

Both looked forward to the evening, the restaurant was attractive, and the food on the menu looked delicious. Jane started to relax, enjoying the quiet music in the background. The waiter took them to their table.

William had barely sat down before he launched in: 'I'll tell you more about my idea for the gift shop by the boatyard. It would be a brilliant place and we know lots of people there already. What do you think? You're right, it's ideal, in the summer there are crowds of visitors, and that means business.'

Jane paused a moment to consider the idea, then opened her mouth to speak, 'I . . .'

'That's just it', said William, 'There may be a few snags, like getting the finance, but we can sort that out. In no time we could be making a profit and getting a good income. We already know a number of manufacturers we can buy from. You feel it's a good idea, don't you?'

Jane pauses again before speaking, 'I'm not sure . . .'

'Not sure about what?' continued William. 'We could run the shop between us, taking it in turns to take the children to school and meet them. It would be simple and we would work well together. What could go wrong?'

The conversation continued like this for most of the meal. William hardly gave Jane a chance to speak, and Jane, who needed to think before speaking, was unable to grasp the little chance she had. Only when they were having coffee did Jane come out with her true reactions to the idea.

'I really feel we ought to wait a few months before rushing into this project. We depend on the income from your present job, and if you gave that up how would we all manage? Also, my part-time job brings in a bit of extra money, so I'd either have to give this up, or if I kept it on I wouldn't be able to help in the gift shop. I feel there are a number of problems we should look at before deciding'.

This speech absolutely amazed William, as Jane had hardly spoken throughout the meal. 'Why on earth didn't you say this earlier? You've had all evening, and you've not said a word. You've had plenty of opportunity. Why did you let me get enthusiastic about the idea if you had reservations?'

Afterwards William felt it was typical of Jane to withhold her thoughts, and Jane felt she was never ever given the space she needed to reflect on what had been said before William was talking his head off again. Both of them had looked forward to the evening out together, but the evening had been spoilt by miscommunication.

When one of us is an E and the other an I in a partnership the E is likely to do more of the talking. Extraverts are re-energized by interaction with other people, and when they are with an I who does not respond immediately they redouble their efforts and talk even more. Introverts need time on their own, or at least to be quiet, to be re-energized. If an E talks and talks they protect themselves by withdrawing.

Sensing and iNtuition (S and N)

Here we have the most interesting and also the greatest difference in preferences between partners. And this difference can cause us agonizing and incomprehensible misunderstandings. We have already seen that we take in information in different ways. Sensing types take in the real and the actual; N types take in impressions, patterns and connections rather than the details. We have seen, too, that we make our subsequent judgements and decisions on different information. It is not difficult to see that two people living in close proximity who differ on S and N are likely to have major misunderstandings: they observe and notice different things and they act on different information. One of the main differences is the way Ss and Ns describe people and events to one another. When going out to the theatre or a function together, for example, they will experience the outing in dissimilar ways. In talking to one another afterwards it is as if they have been to different occasions! And in telling someone else about the occasion Ss start at the beginning, giving the details of how things, looked, smelt, sounded, tasted and felt, whereas Ns describe the occasion by leaping in anywhere, often omitting the supporting details.

All this can bring excitement and a wider dimension to each partner's life, but unless it is understood it can also bring a lot of heartache and sorrow.

John and Emma live in a large market town in the Midlands. John is an S, an IS, and Emma is an N, an EN. Every Wednesday John goes to the Rotary Club lunch. Most of the town's businessmen belong and the local commercial news is exchanged at the Club luncheon. When he comes home in the evening Emma says: 'Meet anyone interesting at the Rotary lunch?'

'I sat next to John Smith today', replies John. 'He is the product manager at Johnson Bros in Green Street. Johnson Bros are moving their offices to Brownlow Street.' Emma looks at him, expecting further information, but doesn't get it. 'I said *interesting*', she says.

'That *is* interesting news', says John. 'Johnson Bros are one of the town's main businesses.' Emma shrugs her shoulders and leaves the room in a huff; John cannot imagine why, as he had tried to give her factual information.

Emma would have responded better if he had said something like, 'I sat next to John Smith, the man with the crooked nose, and he told me that Johnson Bros, the company next door to that funny arch near the station, is moving to those pale green buildings in Brownlow St.' This satisfies Emma's curiosity for patterns and connections, and she can guess the bits that have been omitted. Plain facts make Emma feel she never hears any interesting news from her partner.

And when Emma, as an N, talks to John she gives him few facts, and may omit the step-by-step details which he needs in order to follow her story. John feels Emma's mind flips about and does not stay with the subject. When John, as an S, hears about people and events he likes to be given names, job titles, places and addresses.

Another couple, Jonathan and Jennie, are the reverse, Jonathan being an N and Jennie an S. Jonathan is in the advertising world, and is very creative and imaginative. Jennie runs their large house and is a most capable lady, being very down-to-earth and practical. Jonathan spends most of his working hours thinking in abstract terms, and his mind is rarely centred on the home, and he notices very little in it.

Jennie's mind is centred on the home much of the day, she observes the small practical details in it and sees to these when they need attention.

After they have finished their meal one evening Jennie remarks:

'The border of the carpet in the dining-room is wearing. What do you suggest we do about it?'

Jonathan had never noticed the state of the border of the dining-room carpet, he'd barely noticed the carpet! In his mind he had an impression of the dining-room rather than visualizing it with all the details. He replies, 'I'm not sure what part of the carpet you mean. I haven't noticed anything wrong with it.'

Jennie presumes he notices exactly what she does, and says, 'You cuckoo, can't you see the greek border design is faded and wearing thin?'

'No, I can't', he replies, a bit sheepishly. Jonathan peers at the carpet, and eventually notices that part of it has worn thin.

Jennie is mystified when Jonathan fails to notice the practical details in their home; it is second nature to her to do this. She knows, too, what needs to be done to mend and repair things, and cannot understand it when Jonathan cannot get himself down to these practical details.

But when he starts talking about his ideas and concepts for his advertising brief it is Jennie's turn not to understand. Ideas and concepts make little sense to Ss unless they can be seen to produce specific practical results.

Jennie's practical abilities are appreciated by Jonathan, who openly says he 'does not know what he would do without her', and Jennie says, 'I just don't understand him, I don't think I will ever understand him, but I do love him'.

Jennie is quite right in saying she may never understand how Jonathan takes in information, as it is almost impossible for Ss and Ns to understand how the other's mind works.

It is a good start to be aware that the two methods of collecting information are dissimilar. If we are different from our partner on S and N we will not be surprised or disappointed if we do not expect to observe and experience things in similar ways.

Thinking and Feeling (T and F)

We can find our differences on T and F easier to live with than some of the other preferences. It is more often the expectations of society that cause confusion to partners. Since we have more T males and more F females in society, there is an expectation that men are logical, cool-headed and impersonal, whereas women are more concerned with harmony and understanding personal convictions.

The following conversation takes place one evening when Roger, a T male and his wife Jane, an F female, have some friends round to

111

supper. Married less than two years, each of them is having some difficulty in understanding how the other makes their decisions.

Roger looks at his friend Tony, and says, 'I'd never make decisions using Jane's type of logic – to start with she hasn't got any! She's a typical female, always uses her heart rather than her head.' Tony, also a T, smiles and nods in agreement.

Jane turns towards her friend Sarah, who shares her F preference, and says, 'I feel Roger never takes my feelings into account, he just dismisses them. He's a typical man, always uses his head rather than his heart.' This time Sarah smiles and nods in agreement.

Both Roger and Jane, and Tony and Sarah come to accept their partner's way with a wry smile, all of them feeling their characteristics are typical of their sex.

But the following conversation, between Vera, a successful T businesswoman and Richard, her more gentle F partner, goes against the expectation of society, putting the situation in reverse. Vera feels people are always pushing Richard around, getting him to do the jobs no one else wants to do. When the phone rings again, and it is one of the committee members from the community centre at which Richard helps in his spare time, Vera bristles.

She moans: 'I wish you wouldn't be at the beck and call of the committee members. I certainly wouldn't be. One of them only has to phone, and you stop everything and dash off to do what they want. Who's running your life, you or them?' Vera feels very strongly about this, and speaks aggressively.

A slightly sheepish smile is on Richard's lips, but he says quietly: 'I like to fit in where I can and help people. It won't upset me to do a bit of extra work this evening.' Richard feels it is his responsibility to help people when he can.

But Vera feels her partner is pushed around by others and that he lacks backbone. Richard feels she can be hard and unhelpful, sometimes even unfeminine.

Both Vera and Richard are conscious that they swim against the expectations of society, in spite of the fact that recent years have seen some changes in people's values. In theory we encourage men to exhibit more F behaviour, and to share in childcare and domestic maintenance. Similarly, we encourage women to take up virtually any work they want, and to demonstrate some assertiveness. This makes things easier for the T female and the F male; it seems both are now free to follow their true choices. Yet there is often resentment from the majority of 'typical' T males and F females. Happy in their natural preference, which society has previously affirmed, many of them feel threatened by anything that might upset this.

But, whatever our partner's preference, Ts can put across the need for logic and rational thought, and Fs can put across the need for co-operation and harmony.

Judging and Perceiving (J and P)

At the beginning of a relationship Js and Ps get along most happily. The more rigid and organized J is delighted to find a partner who brings some fun and spontaneity to the relationship. The P, who may long to be more organized and better at managing time, is thrilled to find someone who is able to make plans and keep to schedules. All goes well for a while.

But before long, the J discovers he or she is having to be timekeeper for both of them, and when plans are made which are fixed and settled in the J's view, the P is frequently either late or wants to change the plans at the last minute. And the P soon discovers that his or her freedom is curtailed, and the J insists on knowing times and fixing plans, and this makes the P feel trapped and bound – something Ps dislike intensely. Here we have an area where different preferences can cause tremendous tensions in a partnership.

David and Rebecca live in the country near to a large town, and demonstrate type differences to perfection; both have very strong preferences, David's being P and Rebecca's being J. Rebecca has charge of the home and family, which she loves, and this gives gives her daily, even hourly, opportunities to organize, arrange appointments and see everyone is in the right place at the right time. David, who is also an N, lives in his imagination, dreaming up possible solutions to the world's problems. It is rare for him to be really grounded in the present moment, he has little sense of time, and the needs and practicalities of the home and family life pass him by. Rebecca soon found out David was late for every appointment, as he only started to get ready to go out when the time of the appointment arrived. This infuriated her, and they had row after row. It came to a head one Saturday morning.

'You know your appointment is for 11, you'll be late *again* for the dentist, David', Rebecca shouted.

David, making little effort to hurry, responded, 'I'll get there, what's a few minutes here and there?'

Rebecca knew it would be more than a few minutes; she boiled over inside and felt furious with him. Later that day she wondered what she could do. The next time he had a dental appointment for 11.00 she told him the appointment was for 10.30.

'David, it's nearly 10.30, time to leave for your dental appointment.'

'Just getting ready, we can be off soon', he replied.

'OK. Off we go', agrees Rebecca. She winks at her teenage daughter as they go out, knowing they will be on time. Since then she always tells him the appointment is half-an-hour earlier than it is, he arrives on time and everyone is happy!

Another J and P couple are the other way round, Tom is the J and Gilly is the P. Both of them enjoy going up to art exhibitions in London. When they are thinking about going they get the Sunday newspapers and read as much as they can about the various current exhibitions. Gilly's P mind is then saturated with information and she finds herself unable to decide, not wishing to curtail her options. On her own she would be happy to wait until she arrived in London, and then make up her mind. But her J partner needs to make definite decisions.

'What fun it is looking at the papers this month, there's so much to read and think about', remarks Gilly.

'There is', responds Tom, 'Now we need to make a choice. It's easy to sort out which ones we don't want to visit. That leaves us just the Royal Academy and the Mall Galleries'.

Gilly sighs, 'Why do we have to decide now which ones we'll go to? We're not going until next week. Let's leave it until then.'

'We must decide now and get things settled', Tom replies. 'If we catch the 8.40 train we can go to the Academy in the morning, have lunch at the restaurant there, visit the Mall Galleries in the afternoon, and catch the 4.30 home.'

In order to get a decision Tom has decided for both of them, not just the exhibition they will visit but the times of the trains and where they will have lunch. He feels better once he has made the arrangements for the day, but Gilly feels she has been forced into making choices prematurely.

Strong Js, of which there are plenty, and strong Ps invariably have a hard time getting on together. The Js need for closure and the Ps need to leave things open are opposing. Equally, the Js feel insecure without a structure and the Ps feel trapped within one. It usually works out that the J becomes the timekeeper for the two of them and also arranges any events for them both. Many Js are happy to do this and Ps are happy to have this done for them.

When we look at our different preferences we can see they may both attract and repel us, but at the beginning of a relationship differences frequently attract. Research tells us that without an understanding of type we may know a person for a considerable amount of time before we become fully aware of our differences. We do not know why this is, and this is where our understanding of type can help us. If we are aware of the type of a potential partner at an early stage in the relationship we can be spared many conflicts and misunderstandings.

As well as being aware of the different type preferences we can look at the attraction of different temperaments.

Do temperaments attract?

We have already seen that each of the four temperaments function in a unique and clearly defined manner, and this stems from their needing different things to fulfil what they want in life. These needs and wants are seen as much in our relationships with our partner as in anything else in our lives. As we look at the different temperaments in partners we see specific and identifiable attitudes and behaviour. This gives us considerable help in predicting what is likely to happen between partners of a particular type and temperament.

Here are descriptions of the four temperaments which give us some of the ways each temperament thinks, feels and acts as a partner.

INtuitive–Feeling (NF) temperament

NFs, whether they are male or female, are romantics. They believe in love and all the accompanying qualities that go with this. Affection, tenderness and warmth are important to NFs, and their belief in a romantic partner has a fairy-tale quality to it. Other temperaments may feel romance is the stuff of fiction, but for NFs it is something real and possible. NFs hope that one day they will meet their Prince or Princess and live happily ever after.

These feelings are fuelled by the NF imagination, which is rich and fertile; and when NFs find a partner they feel sure this is the love story of the century. NF lives are permeated with feelings of adoration and imaginative longings. They go out of their way to please their partners, possibly writing love letters with hidden sentimental messages. Other temperaments may not value or understand this behaviour, and if the relationship falls apart NFs are devastated.

NFs have high standards and look for a partner who comes up to these. NFs long for meaning in their lives and seek this through their day-to-day friendships, but above all through their intimate relationship with their partner. But the mundane and tedious details involved in everyday living with their partner seldom comes up to their idealistic expectations. And as the S and T functions may not be well developed, this may leave NFs less secure with the practical realities of this world. Someone who is at home in the concrete world may attract NFs, and may provide them with the necessary grounded qualities needed for daily life, but NFs may end up being bitterly disappointed to discover that this person has little or no comprehension of their world, the world of true love and idealism.

Sex is never a purely physical and functional activity for NFs, it is surrounded by fanciful and shadowy notions of love. The *idea* of sex is more real to them than the act itself; and the mechanics of sex are unlikely to interest them, which may annoy a partner of another temperament. It is the feeling of intimacy and perfect love that matters to them.

INtuitive–Thinking (NT) temperament

The NF temperament may live in the world of romantic idealism, but the NT temperament is more analytical about relationships. NTs are likely to think carefully and rationally – especially the INTs – about their choice of partner. For you everything must be done logically, and that includes selecting a partner. NTs may even make lists, plans or diagrams to work out the pros and cons of a relationship!

The NT way of standing outside a relationship may baffle other temperaments, particularly those with an F preference who invariably feel personally involved in any relationship or situation: partners may feel NTs are oblivious of their feelings, and on occasions oblivious of their presence. There are certainly times when NTs are removed from the present moment – but it may be a moment that is of deep importance to their partner.

Again, NTs may feel deeply about their partner but may not express this to them very often. Having expressed their commitment at the beginning of the relationship NTs are unlikely to repeat it regularly. Other temperaments may feel they need the repeated reassurance of their partner's love and commitment, and may conclude it has been withdrawn.

The NT's partner, if not an NT, may find NTs complex to understand. A female NT may have some difficulty finding a partner with an equally independent lifestyle, allowing her freedom to forge ahead with her own work and interests.

All NTs tend to form their own code of morality which may not be the same as the society they live in. But they believe in and stick to their own morals, seldom swayed by general opinion.

Partners of other temperaments may not find them very interested in domesticity or family occasions. Activities involving fun do not hold much attraction for them either, as they tend to be rather serious with their partners.

NTs desire intellectual discussion and stimulation, and this needs to be understood by their partners. The cut and thrust of an objective discussion or argument can serve as a prelude to sex for NTs. No other temperament is like this and others may find this puzzling. And like the NF, imagination plays an important part for NTs in sex, but they may understand the mechanics better. If NTs are stressed at work or their partner becomes overemotional this can turn NTs off.

Sensing–Judging (SJ) temperament

This is the temperament that is made for a stable and productive partnership. SJs expect their relationships to be ones in which both partners contribute to making a home, and from which they can do something practical and useful for the community. It comes as a surprise to them, therefore, that other temperaments have different goals.

At work SJs are the organizers, the ones who remember appointments and see to details. SJs are the same with their partners. A well-ordered home is important to them and they expect their partners to feel the same. SJs seldom complain about the routines involved in maintaining the home, and expect to fulfil their domestic humdrum chores as part of realistic living.

Although SJs are stable themselves, they are frequently attracted to more exciting, adventurous types. They act as well-grounded and steadfast bases for them. But SJs may find that they are thrown into a shared life of surprise and uncertainty. This can bring fun and new experiences to the SJ but maybe also anxiety and misfortune. It is rare for SJs to walk out on their partner without a very good reason, but not unusual for them to lose their head over an unstable but attractive person.

In recent years, society's expectation of the faithful and permanent couple settling down to create their family unit has been thrown adrift. This is particularly perplexing for SJs, as they need the security of order and permanence with their partners.

Sex is an accepted part of their relationship with their partner. If, for some reason, their partner does not initiate this, SJs may worry, feeling that sex is part of their responsibility and obligation. Unlike the NT, who is put off sex when stressed, SJs see sex as something which brings relaxation when tired or stressed. All Js tend to schedule sex, and SJs in particular are likely to plan this into the weekly activities. Being down-to-earth SJs are probably well acquainted with the details of the physique of both male and female, and prefer it when sex fits in with established routines.

Sensing–Perceiving (SP) temperament

In a long-term relationship partners of other temperaments may have difficulty in understanding SPs, as SPs are many-faceted, and this is likely to appear complex to others. In reality, the SP attitude to life and the actions they choose are comparatively straightforward.

Unlike the NF who looks for romantic love, the NT who analyses relationships, and the SJ who looks to build on ongoing stability, SPs are attracted to what is available at the present moment. Partners may be chosen because they are accessible and obtainable here and now. Tomorrow is rarely thought of, and SPs make the best of today. People of other temperaments are often attracted to SPs, particularly if they are an E, as then their friendliness and open qualities come straight across. Later on others may be surprised to find that SPs are not necessarily interested in continuing to see them, as the next day, week or month takes the SP into new situations. The new situations may or may not include someone s/he was friendly with today.

If they do decide to take a long-term partner, SPs may make a decision about this quite suddenly. Once they have made this decision they will carry it through as quickly as possible, and the chosen person may be swept off his/her feet. If SPs choose a similar partner this allows them both to continue happily and cheerfully, with each day bringing them the possibility of both good and bad fortune.

A partner of another temperament, however, is in for a bit of a shock, especially if they are a J type. When SPs are choosing a long-term partner, a great many choose J partners. They are attracted to their controlled and organized lives, and are happy for them to organize theirs too. But it is not long before SPs begin to feel trapped and tied down as the J's need for order and routine contrasts with the SP need for freedom. The opposing needs pull each of them in different directions.

As partners, SPs can be fun; life is never boring with SPs. SPs seldom look too far ahead or make provision for the future – a characteristic that is unnerving for some types. The SP unpredictability at home and at work may lead to financial instability: one month there is plenty of money – which is likely to be spent, often sharing this generously with their partner – and the next month there is none. Being a light-hearted optimist this does not worry SPs unduly, but it may seriously worry their partner.

SPs are sexually aroused by sensory stimuli – things they see, hear, smell, taste or touch. The symbolic and imaginative world of INtuition means little or nothing to SPs. SPs experience sex as something concrete, and they may talk about sex in a way that others consider vulgar or uncouth, while the variety they like in life extends to liking variety in their sex life.

Summary

If we have more preferences in common with our partner we are likely to experience less conflict and more harmony. But this may lead us to a more confined and limited life, as neither of us may bring anything new to the relationship, and we may both fall short in similar areas.

If both of us are strong SJs, we may work on each other's characteristics of practical, routine hard work, and these become doubled. The house is perfect, the routine may become more rigid and little excitement or new ideas come into our home. Instead of our lives being enriched by each other our lives may become more narrow. Of course this does not need to happen, and a similar way of life can be lived in a more constructive manner. Both of us can have a good understanding of what our partner needs and we can support each other in all we do. We can live and work with little conflict and therefore can achieve what we want without difficulty.

If we choose a partner of a different type or temperament we can be sure each of us brings a contrasting attitude to the partnership. We may have more difficulty in communicating what we need to our partner, and may use up a lot of energy in doing this. And our partner may have little understanding of our needs in life. This may create anxiety, clashes and excursions into unfamiliar territory, but it also gives us variety, excitement and enlarged horizons.

From all this we can see that we provide our partner with the benefits of the characteristics which come easily to us, and we can do no more than this. They provide us with the benefits of *their* characteristics, and it is unrealistic of us to expect them to provide more.

Research tells us that those of us who are aware of our own and our partner's type and temperament have a more solid base on which to build our relationship, as we are more likely to have our partnership anchored in reality.

11
How We Present Ourselves

This chapter shows a different method of looking at the four functions, and gives some important information about Introverts. The method shows that type responds to information and situations in an ordered manner, and goes on to show the order for each type. In the next chapter you can use this knowledge to help you develop aspects of your type.

To make good use of this section you need to know your type. But if you feel unsure of any of your preferences you may be able to use this chapter to help you.

Start by looking at the eight preferences:

Extraversion	**Sensing**	**Thinking**	**Judging**
and	and	and	and
Introversion	**INtuition**	**Feeling**	**Perceiving**

The first pair and the last pair are called *attitudes*. The first pair (Extraversion–Introversion) tell you whether you prefer an outer attitude to the world or an inner attitude to the world. The last pair (Judging–Perceiving) tell you whether your attitude to life is more organized and structured or more flexible and adaptable.

This leaves the two middle pairs. These pairs are called *functions*. They tell you how you *function* in life – how you take in information and how you act on that information.

In previous chapters we have seen how these functions of Sensing and iNtuition, and Thinking and Feeling work in all types. Now we are going to have a special look at the four functions, as they operate in an interesting manner.

These are the four functions:

$$\begin{array}{cc} \textbf{SENSING} & \textbf{THINKING} \\ \updownarrow & \updownarrow \\ \textbf{INTUITION} & \textbf{FEELING} \end{array}$$

You already know that two of these functions are better developed in you than the other two. You know, for example, that if you are an ESTJ type then Sensing and Thinking are better developed in you, and that if you are an INFP type then iNtuition and Feeling are better developed in you.

Of your two better developed functions, one is stronger than the other. This is your *very best function*, your *number one function*. This is the function that responds first to new information or new situations, and it is your most reliable function. After this your number two function responds, backing up your number one. Your third and fourth functions, which you already know to be less developed, can be reached with more difficulty, but they are available.

It is important to understand that our functions respond to the world around us in an *order*: number one coming first, followed by number two, then number three and finally number four. Our number one function, being the best developed, is the one we are most comfortable with. It is also our most reliable and superior function, and it dominates and takes charge of our other functions. For this reason it is called the *dominant function*. Because we are most comfortable with it we try to use it on all occasions. We also feel comfortable using our number two function to back this up, and the two together give us our balance of perception and judgement.

When we need the functions which are less developed in us we usually experience some difficulty in reaching them. They are there, but our best developed functions – being stronger – have already jumped in and made their perceptions and judgements. This makes it much harder for the weaker functions to get a look in. Because we use these less frequently we can experience some difficulty when we do, and we may feel ill-at-ease in using them as they are unfamiliar.

Once you know your number one function you can work out the order of the other three. This chapter is quite complex, however, and you may prefer to go straight to the Table later in this chapter (see p. 127), as this gives the order for each of the 16 types. But if you are interested to look at our diagram on the next page you can learn how to work out the order for yourself.

For example, if Sensing is your number one function, and this is supported by Thinking as your number two function, then Feeling is your number three function and iNtuition is your number four. How can we know this? We know because your number one function (your best developed function) has your least developed function opposite it. If Sensing is your number one and Thinking is your number two, we can work out that Feeling is your number three since iNtuition (being opposite to Sensing) is your number four.

Once we realize that type has a natural order in which the four functions operate, we can understand our reactions to things, and see even more clearly why some of us find some things easy and others more difficult. In time, you can become conscious of the way in which your functions work – and especially conscious of the way in which your number one function takes control of your life.

You might ask why it is that the functions do not operate equally; and would it not be better if they did? From reading previous chapters it is evident that the four functions are opposite ways of living; they are diametrically opposed to one other. If you want to develop your number one function you need to allow it to be used to the full, and this is not possible if it is fighting with its opposite.

But how do we know which is our number one function? We took Sensing as our example, but it could be iNtuition, or Thinking or Feeling.

If you use the diagram and explanation below you can work out your dominant function (and those of other people). This is somewhat like going on a trail in the woods, and you have to be careful to follow the right path to find your number one function. It is worth doing this to get a clear idea of how your functions work in you in different ways. As you follow the arrows be sure you always choose the letters that are part of your type.

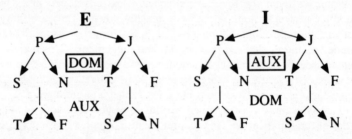

Depending on whether you are E or I you find your *dominant function* in a different way. With Es, their best function is out in the open and they come straight across with it; the function is outside and everyone can see it. With Is, their best function is inside, hidden and not open to all. Few people see the I's best function. After learning to use these diagrams we will look into the way an I functions.

Locating your number one function

Extraverts

To find the E's number one function follow the arrows on the left-hand diagram. Follow the arrow from E to either P or J, whichever is part of the E's type. For an ESTJ follow the arrow to J, and for an ENTP follow the arrow to P. This leads on to S or N, or T or F. For an ESTJ follow the arrow leading to T, and for an ENTP follow the arrow leading to N. This gives their dominant function, giving T for the ESTJ and N for the ENTP.

To go on to find the E's number two, or *auxiliary* function, follow the arrows down to S or N, or T or F. For the ESTJ this leads to S; for the ENTP to T. We know now that the ESTJ number one function is T and that their number two function is S; the ENTP number one function is N and their number two function is T. Note that an E's number two function is inside them, and therefore it is less evident to others. However, since Es are outgoing people they are likely to reveal their number two function by using it openly as they talk. But there are times when we are surprised at things Es may say, and this can be because the thoughts come from their number two function, which is inside.

With the help of the funciton diagram opposite you can work out the third and fourth functions of these types. For the ESTJ, T is the number one function, therefore F (opposite T) is the least developed function, number four; similarly S is the number two function, therefore N is the third function.

For the ENTP, N is the number one function, therefore S (opposite N) is the least developed function, number four; T is the number two function, therefore F is the third function.

Introverts

To find the dominant function for Is, use the right-hand diagram and follow the arrow from I to either P or J, whichever is part of your type. For an INFJ go to the J arrow, and for an ISFP go to the P arrow. This leads on to S or N, T or F. For an INFJ we choose the arrow leading to F, and for an ISFP we choose the arrow leading to S. This gives us their auxiliary function, giving us F for the INFJ and S for the ISFP.

When using this process with Es, their number one function is located; but with Is this gives their number two function – i.e. their supporting or auxiliary function. To find the I's number one function continue to follow the arrow down to S or N, T or F. For the INFJ this leads to N; for the ISFP, to F. So, the INFJ's number one function is N and the number two function is F; for the ISFP, the number one function is F and the number two function is S. The third and fourth functions are found in the same way as with the Es, the fourth being opposite number one and the third being opposite number two.

The difference between Extraverts and Introverts

Following this process may seem long-winded, but it is of special importance in understanding the difference between Es and Is. Look at the diagram again; there is a circle round the *dominant* function for Es and round the *auxiliary* function for Is. This shows which function Es and Is use in their day-to-day dealings with the world. Extraverts are open in showing their dominant function – this can be observed fairly quickly after meeting them. When we meet an ESTJ it is not long before we become aware that they have a logical and objective mind – their number one function (T) is evident to us all. When we meet an ENTP it is not long before we become aware that they flow out with a mass of ideas and possibilities – again their number one function (N) is evident to us all. In many ways this is beneficial all round, the E tells us what he or she knows or proposes, thinks or feels, and we know where we are with them.

With Is, the situation is very different. Is *use their number two function in their day-to-day dealings with the world around them, and their very best function is inside.* This may sound confusing – and it does in fact cause considerable confusion both to the Is themselves and to others. Let's look at what happens.

When we meet an INFJ we meet the number two function, which is F, and often even this is put forward in a reserved manner. We meet someone who shows consideration and understanding for others (F) and frequently we never glimpse his/her very best function, which is N; the INFJ has a mass of ideas and possibilities going round in his/her mind that may not be shared with others.

When we meet an ISFP we meet the number two function first, which is S. We meet someone who shows us his/her commonsense side and sees to practical details. If we do not know the person well we may never be aware of the number one function, F, which is the deep feeling that is frequently the motive that drives them to do these things.

The important thing to remember is that when we meet an I we meet his/her number two function. This is the supporting function, yet because Is use this to deal with the outside world we take this to be their best function, their number one. Introverts are clearly at a disadvantage, as people are unaware of their number one function as it is hidden. Friends, colleagues and even family are also at a disadvantage as they usually have to deal with the I without having access to his/her best function. It is not surprising that judgements are made about Is which are rarely based on a full knowledge of them.

Following the procedure above, this helps to see why the I's number one function is inside and hidden. Now you understand this, we can look at another method of finding your number one function, and some of you may find this method simpler.

Finding your number one function: method 2

Note whether your type is P or J. This tells you which of your functions you use in dealing with the outside world. If you are P, you use your Perceiving function (S or N); if you are J, you use your Judging function (T or F).

As an ESTJ is a J, s/he uses the Judging function (T) to deal with the outside world; since s/he is an E this is the number one function. But an ISTJ, also J, uses the Judging function (T) to deal with the outside world too; but, as an I, this is the number two function, and the number one function is inside, and this is S.

As an ENFP is a P, s/he uses the Perceiving function (N) in the outside world; since s/he is an E this is the number one function. But an INFP, also P, uses the Perceiving function (N) in the outside world too; but, as an I, this is the number two function and the number one function, F, is inside.

The following story shows how our number one function dominates our immediate response to new information.

It was Saturday afternoon on an August Bank Holiday weekend at the local tennis club, and a mixed doubles had just finished. Another member came up to the four players, and said:

'Would you all be interested in playing at the Waterside Club on Monday?'

Completely different thoughts came into the minds of the four players.

The player whose number one function was S thought: 'None of us has a car, so how will we all get there? It will mean using public transport, which may not be running on a Bank Holiday; and how will we get home again?'

The player whose number one function was N thought: 'Wonderful idea. Large airy grounds, and a huge club house.' Visions of immaculate grass courts bathed in sunshine came into his mind.

The player whose number one function was T thought: 'Sounds more trouble than it's worth. With five of us there'll be a hassle over who sits out. Don't think I want to be involved.'

And the player whose number one function was F thought: 'There's five of us, someone is going to be left out; Oh dear', feeling suddenly pained at this inevitable prospect.

The responses above tell us the players' immediate thoughts on hearing the same remark. Of course they all thought further about the suggestion, and other things came into their minds, but our number one function is so strong it dominates the thoughts which follow and makes them fit in with it.

Stretching your other functions

It is not difficult to see that all of us have times in our lives when we could make use of a different, more appropriate, dominant function. It would be handy to be able to do this by just calling it up! But we do not work like this, and the number one function will always dominate the others. However, you can learn to stretch your use of the functions by making deliberate use of all of them. In this way, decisions and opinions can be better considered and more balanced.

Choose a situation in your life which you would like to see from a wider perspective and from a different angle. It can be something quite small and apparently unimportant as most situations respond to this method.

First make use of your S and N functions to be aware of how you notice and perceive people and things in this situation. Use your S first (even if it happens to be your fourth and least developed function) to try and look at the situation realistically, noting as many facts as you can, telling yourself what the present situation is and being aware of what you and other people are doing now. If this is difficult try to describe the situation as if you were an outside observer reporting facts.

Go on to use your N to look at ways you might change the situation, or change aspects of the situation. Could other people's attitudes be changed? Are there any other things you could change?

Next, use your T to look at the situation in an impersonal manner, as an outside observer. Consider any possible solutions, and think what the consequences of each of these might be. Take into account the benefits of any solutions you dislike.

Finally, use your F to consider how much you care about the outcome – in particular, the long-term outcome. Look at how other people's lives and emotions will be affected by the different solutions, and take your own and other people's feelings into consideration.

When doing this (which is nothing like as easy as it sounds) you are looking at a situation from a number of perspectives; you are bringing to mind the concrete and factual information; looking at ways you might change things; considering cause and effect, and taking people's feelings into account. In all you are making your decisions on more information. You are still likely to make your decisions using your best developed functions, but by considering many other aspects and perspectives, you are at least making these decisions more balanced.

Below is the list of the 16 types, giving the order in which the functions work. The number one function of the Is is underlined as a reminder that we may miss this because it is hidden.

Type	Function 1	Function 2	Function 3	Function 4
ENFJ	FEELING	INTUITION	SENSING	THINKING
INFJ	<u>INTUITION</u>	FEELING	THINKING	SENSING
ENFP	INTUITION	FEELING	THINKING	SENSING
INFP	<u>FEELING</u>	INTUITION	SENSING	THINKING
ENTJ	THINKING	INTUITION	SENSING	FEELING
INTJ	<u>INTUITION</u>	THINKING	FEELING	SENSING
ENTP	INTUITION	THINKING	FEELING	SENSING
INTP	<u>THINKING</u>	INTUITION	SENSING	FEELING
ESTJ	THINKING	SENSING	INTUITION	FEELING
ISTJ	<u>SENSING</u>	THINKING	FEELING	INTUITION
ESFJ	FEELING	SENSING	INTUITION	THINKING
ISFJ	<u>SENSING</u>	FEELING	THINKING	INTUITION
ESTP	SENSING	THINKING	FEELING	INTUITION
ISTP	<u>THINKING</u>	SENSING	INTUITION	FEELING
ESFP	SENSING	FEELING	THINKING	INTUITION
ISFP	<u>FEELING</u>	SENSING	INTUITION	THINKING

12

Developing Your Shadow

When we first discover our type most of us feel encouraged and affirmed. It is as if someone is saying to us: 'The pattern of your life is right for you, you are fine the way you are. Concentrate on your positive qualities'. It is important for us to feel this, as we need to appreciate the benefits of our type and we need confirmation of our way of living before we can think of expanding and developing ourselves.

None of us would claim that our type is fully developed, but some of us have been fortunate in having a life which has nurtured our type. Some of us have been less fortunate and may feel our development is somewhat stunted. We already know some of the reasons for this. Chapter 9 illustrated how any type that is radically different from other members of a family can be ignored or squashed; a pupil different from a teacher made unhappy at school, never fitting in, and any number of influences may have prevented us from being our true selves. If we are fortunate, we find our own ways of developing our type preferences, and this gives us deep satisfaction. If we are unable to do this we may carry on in life to take up work or a lifestyle that is contrary to our nature, and we always have a sense of dissatisfaction; we are living as a false type. If you feel this, you need to concentrate on becoming fully aware of your own type and temperament, and learn to live this out to the full, rather than striving to develop your opposite preferences. Only when we are stronger in our own type can we think about developing our other side or shadow.

Your attitude to life

Before we go on to see how we might develop our type we can first consider our attitude towards life. Different types have different attitudes to life; they see life in different ways and want different things. NFs look for personal meaning in life; NTs seek intellectual understanding; SJs are here to be useful and do their duty; SPs live for the enjoyment of today.

We can have these different aspirations, but all of us want to make the most of ourselves in order to get the most out of life.

We can help ourselves do this by developing our preferences and also by developing our *shadow*, the part of us that is hidden and undeveloped. Some of us may like to look at this in terms of light and darkness, or personal growth and spiritual development. We can see that the part of us which is better developed – our type – is available for our use. It is as if it is in the light: we are conscious of it and can see it. The part of us which is undeveloped is not yet available for our use, and we are less conscious of these characteristics; we cannot see these as they are still in the dark. One way we can look at this is to think of bringing some of the dark areas across into the light. In terms of type this is to develop aspects of our opposite preferences so that they become part of our conscious life and are available for our use. Our shadow then becomes part of us and is able to support and enrich our type. Those of us who believe we have a spirit within us can see this as working towards our spiritual development.

The idea is not to try turning into our opposite type; this would be inappropriate. We are our own type, but there are times when we become aware that it is helpful to make use of one or more of our opposite preferences. Often this can be immensely difficult and frustrating but we need not feel resentful or stoical when we do this if we remember that we do this to back up and strengthen our type, and therefore it is for the benefit of our type. It may involve some pain, suffering, struggle and conflict but ultimately we extend and enrich our lives. This can be exciting and bring us the reward of deeper happiness and success. By developing aspects of our opposite preferences we are able to have 'more' of ourselves, we become more balanced, rounded and complete. We know when this is happening to us, and other people notice this too.

Getting to know your opposite type

If you are interested to make use of your shadow by developing aspects of your opposite preferences here are some suggestions for doing this.

Start by reading the Profile in Chapter 4 of your opposite type, and form a positive image of this type. You can then imagine someone of this type as s/he might go about her/his normal day. By picturing some of the details of what this person observes, thinks, feels and does, you are able to get some insight into the way this type experiences her/his life. You can also think about what this type finds difficult and what s/he enjoys. Are there particular things about this type that you admire?

And are there situations in your life which might improve if you made use of one or more preferences of this type? Try to consider each preference in turn and see how and where these might be of benefit to you. If we are willing to study our opposite type we can gain some penetrating insights into ourselves; and sometimes this helps us to see why we upset some of the other types.

We are now going to look at the types in turn, and read some of the things which other people find vexing or disturbing about each type. These comments will be put strongly so that they are understood clearly. Most contain more than a grain of truth but they need not necessarily apply personally. Decide which of them are relevant to you.

ENFJ

Some comments made about ENFJs:

'She assumes she knows what everyone wants.'

'He's so talkative and persuasive it's difficult to speak out and disagree with him.'

'She is always rushed.'

'He gets upset very easily if any of us question his judgment.'

'She often forgets the small details because she is dashing off to the next thing.'

To enrich your type:

- Read the ISTP profile.
- Remember to give time to small practical details – your work will benefit.
- Be aware of what is happening in the present instead of rushing on with the next thing.
- Try to be sure you have the necessary facts for any project you are involved in, so that your decisions are more soundly based.
- Try to use more impersonal, logical thought in all areas of your life.
- Listen carefully to what others are saying.
- Give others time to speak and see if sometimes you can adapt to fit in with them.
- Try to spend some time on your own.

INFJ

Some of the comments made about INFJs:

'She is hard to get to know.'

'He is slow to make up his mind, and stubborn about changing it.'

'She leads a restricted life, as she seldom joins in group activities.'

'I have seen him being kind and understanding, but you would never guess this as he comes across as somewhat cool and reserved.'

'She is such a serious person, she misses a lot of fun in life.'

To enrich your type:

- Read the ESTP profile.
- Try to increase your knowledge of the practical world.
- Be more aware of specific things that are taking place around you.
- See if you can develop your logical side by using this in your work and your interests.
- Be willing to adapt to changing circumstances and other people's wishes.
- Try to be more outgoing, and people will enjoy getting to know you.

ENFP

Some of the comments made about ENFPs:

> 'She never sticks at anything for very long.'

> 'He always passes the work on without completing the practical details.'

> 'She loses interest very quickly.'

> 'He's not someone I'd rely on to do the job on a regular basis.'

> 'She just walks off if something disagreeable has to be dealt with.'

To enrich your type:

- Read the ISTJ profile.
- Remember to see to the practical details of your projects.
- Try to see that any task you take on gets finished on time.
- Be sure to keep your word when you make promises and commitments, even small ones.
- Try to leave yourself some personal inner space instead of overloading yourself with numerous activities.
- Make a rational attempt to take stock of your life at home and at work.
- Bring some routine and order into your home and work life.

INFP

Some of the comments made about INFPs:

> 'She's a wanderer, with little focus to her life.'

> 'He's not rooted in the real world.'

> 'How can we employ her, she's neither organized nor down-to-earth.'

> 'He's not got the drive to push this project through.'

> 'She lives in her own world, going round in circles, getting nowhere.'

To enrich your type:

- Read the ESTJ profile.
- Attempt the small practical tasks necessary for daily living.
- Become aware of time and make a habit of being punctual.
- Try to go out to others as too much privacy may mean you become introspective.
- Listen to others' thoughts and feelings and be willing to share some of your deeper emotions.
- In your home and social life try sometimes to be the one who sees to the practical needs of the moment.
- Be willing to enforce your opinion if you feel strongly about something.

ENTJ

Some of the comments that are made about the ENTJs:

'He doesn't listen to other people's views.'

'She's bossy and overbearing.'

'He goes ahead without checking the practical details of the scheme.'

'Once she's made her mind up she'll never change it.'

'He's like a sergeant major, even at home.'

To enrich your type:

- Read the ISFP profile.
- Keep your mind on what is going on at the moment.
- Remember to see to the step-by-step factual details.
- Try developing an artistic hobby is beneficial as this brings you relaxation, which is difficult for your type.
- Try to build an awareness of the natural world and its beauty.
- Go with the flow of life sometimes, it will help you to be more adaptable and flexible.
- Encourage others to share their feelings with you, and be willing to share your own.

INTJ

Some of the comments made about INTJs:

'He's a very cold fish.'

'She's a loner and doesn't seem to need anyone.'

'He may have some good ideas, but he's so arrogant.'

'She never laughs and jokes.'

'He thinks he's the only one who knows anything.'

To enrich your type:

- Read the ESFP profile.
- Try listening to others' opinions and suggestions, and value these; it will help you to work with others better.
- Try to be aware of the more concrete details of the world around you.
- Become aware of the importance of people's needs on a practical daily basis.
- Try to develop a warm and friendly manner to people: they'll respond to you.
- Be willing to get involved in small matters at work, home or your community.
- Try to have some fun!

ENTP

Some of the comments made about ENTPs:

'He's such a know-all.'

'She's never still for a minute, always on to the next thing.'

'He can't be relied on to do the work behind the scenes, he's got to be upfront.'

'She's always organizing other people to do her work.'

'He's not prepared to sit down quietly and listen to me.'

To enrich your type:

- Read the ISFJ profile.
- Be prepared to stay quietly in the background and listen to others, you will understand a situation better.
- Be sure you see to the small practical and factual details of projects.
- Carry projects right through to the end.
- Be willing to see to the needs of those around you rather than rushing off to the next activity.
- Try to take time for yourself to plan some routine into your life.
- Prepare for the tasks you do at home and at work, and clear up after them.

INTP

Some of the comments made about INTPs:

'His ideas are so far-fetched, they never work out in reality.'

'She's just a brain, she's not really in this world.'

'His sense of time is appalling, he's late for everything.'

'She's not an affectionate person.'

'He's not interested in the everyday things of life, he lives in cloud cuckoo land.'

To enrich your type:

- Read the ESFJ profile.
- Try to get involved with the practical day-to-day routine at home or at work; this will help to ground you.
- Listen to others' views, and be willing to consider their views; this might be valuable, and will widen your understanding of life.
- Try to be warm and friendly with those you meet, and considerate of their individual needs.
- See if you can express your deeper feelings to people you know.
- Try to become more aware of time throughout the day.

ESTJ

Some of the comments made about ESTJs:

'He's so domineering, he never listens.'

'She always wants to be in charge.'

'He's always the first with the answer, none of the rest of us get a chance.'

'She puts everything into action before you've had time to consider whether it's the best thing.'

'He never bothers to ask what others think and feel.'

To enrich your type:

- Read the INFP profile.
- Plan to spend some time alone in reflection; this will allow you time to consider your decisions more deeply and less hurriedly.
- Look ahead in your life and your work to see what might happen.
- Picture different situations; try to see that there can be more than one possible outcome and more than one way of tackling projects; someone else's way might be better.
- Try to express warm feelings for those you live and work with, and be willing to adapt your plans to fit in with others.
- If others do something well, be prepared to praise them.

ISTJ

Some of the comments made about ISTJs:

'He comes across as cold and unfeeling.'

'She has little to say, I wouldn't call her an asset at a party.'

'I've tried to draw him out, but he doesn't seem to have much to him.'

'Her conversation is limited to facts in the past, she can't catch on to new ideas.'

'He's set in his ways, absolutely unadaptable.'

To enrich your type:

- Read the ENFP profile.
- Try to show warmth and enthusiasm to others.
- Broaden your experience of different people.
- Try not to dismiss new ideas as impractical.
- See if you can look ahead and plan some small project for the future.
- Spend some time getting involved with something new.
- Be willing to fit in with others and change your plans.
- When someone does something for you let them know that you appreciate this.

ESFJ

Some of the comments made about ESFJs:

'She never stops talking.'

'He's not happy unless he's doing something.'

'She hasn't got an ounce of logic in her.'

'It's hard to get a word in edgeways with him.'

'She can't follow an idea or concept.'

To enrich your type:

- Read the INTP profile.
- Learn to value yourself as an individual.
- Try to spend some time alone rather than living through the practical service you give to others.
- Try to hold back in conversation, you will learn a great deal about how others think, feel and live.
- An IN friend can bring you a way of looking at life that enriches you.
- When people come up with ideas and concepts try not to dismiss them without at least opening your mind to considering them.

135

- Be willing to change your routine occasionally.

ISFJ

Some of the comments made about ISFJs:

'She's a doormat.'

'He's always in the background, he has no ambition.'

'She waits on him hand and foot.'

'He's got no drive or push, he'll never get anywhere.'

'She never speaks out, so we are never sure what she feels.'

To enrich your type:

- Read the ENTP profile.
- Try to be more forceful about matters that are important to you.
- Make yourself more physically and verbally visible rather than going unrecognized in the background.
- Try to start a new interest by yourself.
- Make an effort to look at things as a whole rather than the small details, and this will help you to accept new ideas at home and at work.
- Be willing to speculate about how new ideas for home and work might work out.
- Change or adjust your routine and plans.

ESTP

Some of the comments made about ESTPs:

'He's never there when I need him.'

'She plays to the gallery, I'm not sure when I'm meeting the real person.'

'I can never depend on him to be on time.'

'She's not someone who is good at understanding people.'

'It's hard to explain an idea to him, as he's so caught up with what's going on in the present.'

To enrich your type:

- Read the INFJ profile.
- Listen carefully to others of different types, and be willing to sympathize with them in their troubles.
- Try and show warmth and understanding to those you live and work with.

- Give yourself time to allow your own feelings to surface.
- Try to do some things on your own without needing others to be there.
- Be sure that you see to the details of any project you want to take to completion.
- Be willing to consider more abstract thoughts and ideas.

ISTP

Some of the comments made about ISTPs:

'He doesn't understand my feelings.'

'She wasn't interested in being part of the group, only in what the group was doing.'

'He's pretty cold and calculating.'

'She often doesn't turn up on time.'

'He just went off on his own, oblivious of what the rest of us felt.'

To enrich your type:

- Read the ENFJ profile.
- Make an effort to be warm and friendly to people – they will respond to you, especially if you show sympathy and understanding.
- Try to keep your promises and commitments so that people feel they can depend on you.
- Be willing to discuss others' ideas.
- Look for points of agreement before you dismiss others' ideas as impractical.
- Do not reject your intuition when you have hunches or ideas; instead, allow these to develop, looking for the benefits both for yourself and for others.

ESFP

Some of the comments made about ESFPs:

'She leaps into action before she has thought through the scheme.'

'I can't pin him down.'

'She takes on too many things at the same time, and then can't fulfil them all.'

'He pretends unpleasant things have not happened, and refuses to face up to serious matters.'

'She's always on to the next thing, leaving a number of commitments incomplete.'

To enrich your type:

- Read the INTJ profile.
- Take time alone for yourself away from your usual busy, cheerful and active life.
- Try to think carefully about the numerous things you do, and consider these in a logical and decisive manner.
- Decide whether you want to be involved in all your different activities, or whether you do them just because they are there.
- Try and find out what life means to you.
- Commit yourself to a project which you carry through to completion on your own.
- Be willing to listen to scientific ideas, accepting that some of them can be of practical use.

ISFP

Some of the comments made about ISFPs:

'She's so self-effacing, I never know if I'm meeting the real person.'

'I could not recommend him to represent the company as he's not an upfront person.'

'She gets so involved in the small details of numerous projects, and never has time to devote herself to the main one.'

'He never says much, so I seldom know how he feels about things.'

'She's not forceful enough to be in charge of the team.'

To enrich your type:

- Read the ENTJ profile.
- Try to see the 'big picture' in life rather than always getting involved in minute details.
- Try to take some small position of leadership, and organize a project through to the end.
- Be willing to stick to your opinion in an argument even if others disagree with you.
- You are usually behind the scenes; see if you can sometimes bring yourself forward into the limelight so that others can be aware of your accomplishments.
- Try to see some things from a scientific and logical point of view.

As we read the suggestions above we can remember that all of us are frail human beings, and we need to be realistic in our expectation of ourselves and others. Our lives are different, not only in type, but also in experience. The right time for one person to be thinking of type development may not be the right time for someone else.

In general terms most of us find that our young adult years are preoccupied with choosing and building a career, finding a partner and bringing up a family. During these years we tend to live and work out of our preferences, and it may be middle life before we think about personal or spiritual development. Sometimes we do this at a point of crisis, or we may become aware of other areas of life in which we are drawn to take part.

Trying to make aspects of our shadow part of our conscious self can be rewarding, and give us great satisfaction. We can develop in sudden leaps, but we also find we fall back frequently which makes us disappointed with ourselves. All of us know that we fluctuate in the way we live and often this is due to our current personal circumstances.

We can look at this as living on different levels. When life goes well for us and we produce our best we live at our best. But we cannot stay there all the time, and we need to accept that we have fluctuations in life, which means that our way of living and being goes up and down.

Developing your opposite characteristics

The suggestions given above are some of the ways in which we can try to strengthen our lesser-used characteristics. But there are other ways we can go about developing our shadow. We can take all our opposite preferences, and look at positive ways of making use of these. Below are some suggestions for doing this, and each of us can decide how many of these are helpful to us.

Developing Extraversion for Introverts

You already have some E, which you have developed in order to live in the world.

- Try to be with people one at a time, or in small numbers as crowds may suffocate you.
- You'll find it easier to be with others, if you can become involved in activities which interest you.
- Ask other people about their news and events.
- Try to take your chance in conversations and have your say.
- Be willing to have greater breadth of interest in a number of things rather than depth of interest in a few.
- See that you do not spend too long considering, and possibly miss something by failing to act.

139

- Try to show and communicate your best function to others – remember this is inside and others are not aware of this.
- Keep in touch with what is going on in the outside world, especially if you're an IN.
- Pay attention to interruptions, as these may be important.
- Realize that you can be sociable for a certain amount of time, knowing you can choose when you return into yourself.

Developing Introversion for Extraverts

Extraverts may have developed very little I, and can try to make a friend of silence, even in public.

- Give more time to considering things more deeply and with more concentration.
- Take time to be on your own and listen to yourself, understanding that you have an inner life.
- Find a task or hobby which you enjoy that you can do on your own.
- Build up your one-to-one relationships so that you experience these at greater depth.
- Ask questions of others, and listen carefully to the answers until the person has finished speaking. Try not to jump in with your own thoughts.
- If you are in a group make sure each person has had a chance to speak before you speak again.
- Think carefully before acting, and then act.

Developing Sensing for iNtuitives

- Try to look at the realistic and practical thing to do first, then see if your ideas make sense.
- Be patient when following instruction books, they usually need to be read step-by-step.
- Try to improve your eye for detail, you might compare what you notice with an S friend.
- Accept that established methods of doing things generally work.
- You can learn from the past, as it will usually tell you what has worked well and what has not.
- If you concentrate on staying in the present moment this will allow you to enjoy present pleasures, which you often miss.
- Facts are both important and useful, try to know when you need to make use of them.
- Remember: thinking up something is not the same as doing it!
- Good ideas may come to nothing if you fail to take small and precise details into account.

- If you need to explain your ideas to others you put them across better if you do so in an orderly and matter-of-fact manner.
- As you go around learn to notice signposts and other landmarks.
- See if you can give others full and accurate directions to places.

Developing iNtuition for Sensers

- Try doing a job in an unusual way, it may not work but you are likely to learn something.
- Think of something which is important to you now. Imagine what might happen with this in the future, and try to think of a number of different things. Doing this can help you make better judgements in the present.
- If you have a 'hunch' see if you can follow this up and take some notice of it.
- When looking around you or studying something, try to see the thing as a whole.
- Make an effort to think about something in a conceptual and abstract manner.
- See if you can think ahead and plan something creative for the future. If it is possible try and carry this through to completion.

Developing Thinking for Feelers

- See if you can stand outside and watch a situation instead of feeling involved in it.
- Even if it means disagreeing with someone, stick to your beliefs and convictions.
- Try to look at situations logically and rationally, bringing some objectivity to the situation.
- Be more outspoken with those around you, especially if you are I.
- Try to be less personally concerned in the day-to-day circumstances that occur, many of these may not really involve you.

Developing Feeling for Thinkers

- Before disagreeing with people be sure you consider their opinions and points of view.
- Try to develop some close friendships and be willing to spend time and patience nurturing them.
- Learn to work better with others by being more co-operative and tolerant, they will appreciate this.
- Find ways of giving specific appreciation to others by praising them verbally.
- You can get in touch with your own feelings more if you try and express these to those around you.

- Try not to force your will on others.
- Try not to add to any conflict; try to negotiate and conciliate.
- Consider people's feelings, by giving some warmth, compassion and sympathy when needed. This is logical.
- Listen to others' ideas with enthusiasm and an open mind.

Developing Judging for Perceivers

- Be willing to see to the follow-up details of something that needs your attention.
- Plan and prepare for a project, organize it and carry it through to completion *on time*.
- Decide who or what you are responsible for in specific terms, and carry your responsibilities through.
- Try not to prevaricate when a decision is needed.
- Accept the rules and regulations at work or elsewhere, they may seem unnecessary but others may value them.
- Check that those around you are not put out because you have neglected anything they depend on.
- Make some decisions about the purpose and path of your own life and try to hold on to these.
- Look at the long-term consequences of your present actions or lack of actions.
- Ask yourself regularly if you are being reliable.

Developing Perceiving for Judgers

- Try to keep an open mind about those around you rather than making hasty judgments.
- Be sure you gather as much information as you need before making your decisions.
- Make a point of leaving some unplanned time without organizing anything ahead; when the time arrives see what is happening around you and then decide what to do.
- Keep your mind open to other people's points of view.
- Be willing (if SJ) to try different ways of doing things, other than the standard ones.
- Instead of turning down an opportunity that crops up suddenly act on impulse and accept it.
- Break away from one of your usual routines for a while to see how it feels.
- If things do not turn out as planned try not to worry, and be more adaptable and willing to change your plans.
- See if you can take a risk and be more adventurous.

- See if you can be more relaxed and less rigid, and try to be more flexible with others.

Throughout this book we have looked at type and temperament as they affect us in the most important areas of our lives, and we have seen ways of avoiding pitfalls and ways of enriching our type.

We need to be sensitive to ourselves when we think about developing our type. We can see this as being a life-long attitude rather than something we do now and then. Our type tells us which of our preferences are better developed, but it does not tell us the extent of their development or whether these preferences are developed in positive ways.

We can make it part of our purpose in living to extend the qualities of our type. In doing this we become open to more information about ourselves; and as more information becomes available to us we find we can use this in positive ways for our personal happiness and fulfilment. Everyone else benefits too.

13
Working with Type in Seminars, Conferences and Groups

Although the different characteristics become more and more apparent to us, some of us become curious to experience these differences in a more practical and realistic situation.

A number of seminars and courses are now available to us in different parts of the country, and these are organized by management consultants and psychologists, religious and spiritual groups and other people. We might wonder what happens when we go on one of these courses.

We have the chance of meeting others who are interested in type, and of turning theory into reality. Each course has its own emphasis, but an introductory course is sure to include some basic information about type preferences, and how these relate to us at home, at work and in our social lives. There may be the opportunity of working on a simple project with others who share our preferences, and perhaps with those who are different. If you are interested in going on a course it is best to find out the details of what this covers before you book in.

At my introductory weekends we spend some time hearing about the four pairs of preferences, and as we see and experience these in one another our understanding becomes stronger and firmer. It is give and take – we let others know about us and they let us know about themselves, and we can do this knowing that all the preferences are valuable and positive. Learning what we are *not* is surprisingly helpful too. This gives us a solid base on which we can learn more, and many of us are surprised at how much understanding develops between us.

There are opportunities to be in small groups during the weekend to work with those who share our preferences. We might start by collecting our positive characteristics, and most of us are surprised at the breadth and depth of what we collect together, far more than we would on our own. This encourages everyone in the group. Later, we share our findings with the other groups, and they tell us what they have collected. All of us benefit.

If there is time, or at a follow-on weekend, we look at temperament. Doing simple projects in groups with others who share our temperament gives us a straightforward way of experiencing differences. As we get to know those in our temperament group we are amazed to find how much we have in common.

At a follow-on weekend we have time to look more closely at the four functions and at our dominant function. We might spend time looking at the possible negative characteristics of our type, and how we can avoid these letting us down. Perhaps we work on ways of developing our shadow, and we might look back on our childhood influences. The great advantage of being with others is that we can see and hear about all these characteristics in reality.

Here is the experience of a young woman, Ellen, who became interested to see type in action, and she came to one of my weekend conferences.

During the weekend Ellen found much satisfaction from meeting another female of her type, especially as she was INTJ, an infrequent type for females. The two INTJs discovered they had much in common, not just in interests, but in their attitude to the world and in the specific ways they liked to tackle things in their lives. They were an encouragement to one another, and both of them went home determined to use their strengths more in the future.

Ellen also found it fascinating to meet others who were quite different from her. She did not find her opposite type, which she would have liked, but she met many others who had two or three different preferences from herself. She was able to talk with a number of them and clarify the differences between them. As the weekend progressed people were amazed as more and more differences became apparent, and they all gained much insight into themselves and those around them. When Ellen left on the Sunday afternoon, she described the weekend as 'Mind-blowing!'

Not all of us can get to seminars or weekends and there are other ways of learning more. One of these is by joining a group which meets to enrich their knowledge of type. We might join a group which already exists or we might start our own group. Whatever we do each group becomes unique as it is made up of different people.

Groups need to have a purpose for meeting. This might be for individual or spiritual development – in which case the level of communication is more personal – or it might be to discover more in practical terms how the different types think, feel and act in a variety of situations. You may have your own ideas of why your group should meet.

Here are some suggestions which have been found to help groups work well. A group needs to run smoothly, and to be both useful and creative for its members. Someone needs to be responsible for this and for drawing the best out of everyone. This need not be a leader in the sense of manager, but certainly a facilitator is needed. He or she can see that everyone gets a fair chance of speaking, and that the Is are not left out.

If the general purpose of the group is established, different topics can be chosen for each meeting. You might take one of the pairs of preferences, each person saying how they feel their preference is useful. This often reveals new ways in which we can act, and sometimes this shows us where we fall short. Try looking at all four pairs of preferences in turn. Temperament provides another way of understanding our differences. Other topics might be to describe our ideal work or ideal lifestyle. As we do these things we expand our knowledge of ourselves and others. Members of the group will probably come up with suggestions for a number of topics. If the group continues to meet, an interesting topic might be to look at ways of developing your shadow side.

A group needs some structure and consistency to help it cohere. Without this it becomes like a house with no foundation, and there is no base to build on. Judgers take happily to a structure, but Ps may prefer a less structured approach. One way of sorting this out might be to start by going round the group in turn, giving each person two to three minutes, and then to go round again before opening out the group for free discussion. The facilitator can see that people do not overrun their time. Once we move into discussion we tend to become more generalized, and the Is are likely to get left out. Again, it is the facilitator's task to see that everyone gets a fair chance.

This way there is some structure brought into the group, and this provides a base from which we can move into a less structured time.

Towards the end of the time it is helpful to go over some of the more important things that come up. As with seminars and conference weekends it is often surprising how much we learn about other people, and therefore about ourselves. Some people have a particular gift for facilitating groups, but if members wish, different people can take a turn at this. As far as numbers go, up to 10 or 12 people works well, but the group becomes too big after this and needs to divide into two.

These suggestions are to get you started, and your group will eventually like to organize itself in its own way.

Throughout this book we have looked at type and temperament as they affect us in the most important areas of our lives, and we have seen ways of avoiding pitfalls and ways of enriching each type.

As you continue with your life, determine to be yourself – but be your best self.

Summary of Temperament

INtuitive-Feeling	*Sensing-Judging*
enthusiastic	dependable
humane	factual
religious	painstaking
subjective	routinized
sympathetic	thorough
insightful	conservative
creative	consistent
imaginative	detailed
linguistic	hard-working
research oriented	patient
sensitive	persevering
idealistic	sensible
loyal	stable

INtuitive-Thinking	*Sensing-Perceiving*
abstract	adaptable
analytic	artistic
complex	athletic
curious	realistic
efficient	calm
exacting	easy-going
impersonal	enjoy life
independent	good natured
ingenious	open minded
intellectual	persuasive
inventive	mechanically-minded
logical	tolerant
scientific	un-prejudiced
theoretical	sensitive to colour, line, texture
research oriented	store useful facts
systematic	cheerful

Taken from Keirsey, David. *Portraits of Temperament*. Prometheus Nemesis Book Co. US (1987). Used with permission.

Further Information

The Personality Discovery Questionnaire provides you with a guide to your type and temperament. The disk can be used 50 times, and all the scores are retained for your future reference.

If you would like more information about the disk and/or information about future conferences, please send a large S.A.E. to Patricia Hedges, 52 Entry Hill, Bath, Somerset, BA2 5LU.

The Vision, published annually by The National Retreat Association, lists details of a number of courses of a religious nature on Myers-Briggs, *The Vision* can be obtained from retreat centres and Christian bookshops, or direct from The National Retreat Association at Liddon House, 24 South Audley Street, London W1Y 5DL.

Further Reading

I found the following books particularly useful while writing this book:

Briggs Myers, Isabel. *Gifts Differing*. Consulting Psychologists Press, Inc., Palo Alto, California (1980). Obtainable from Oxford Psychologists Press, 311–321 Banbury Road, Oxford OX2 7JH (tel: 0865 510203). (This book was useful for Chapter 11.)

Golay, Keith. *Learning Patterns and Temperament Styles*. Manas Systems, Newport Beach, California (1982). (I made use of this in Chapter 8.)

Hirsch, Sandra Krebs and Kummerow, Jean M. *Introduction to Type in Organizational Settings*. Consulting Psychologists Press, Inc. (1987). Obtainable from Oxford Psychologists Press (as above).

Keirsey, David. *Portraits of Temperament*. Prometheus Nemesis Book Co. US (1987).

Keirsey, David, and Bates, M. *Please Understand Me: Character and Temperament Types*. Prometheus Nemesis Book Co. US (1978). Obtainable from Oxford Psychologists Press (as above). (These two books formed the basis of the sections on temperament, especially when compiling the descriptions of temperament in Chapter 5 and the Summary of Temperament on page 147.)

Kroeger, Otto and Thuesen, Janet M. *Type Talk: The 16 Personality Types that Determine how we Live, Love and Work*. Obtainable from Oxford Psychologists Press (1988).

Kroeger, Otto and Thuesen, J. *Type Talk at Work*. Tilden Press, Delacorte Press New York (1992). Obtainable from Oxford Psychologists Press (as above).

Michael, C. and Norrisey, M. *Prayer and Temperament*. The Open Door Inc., PO Box 855 Charlottesville, Virginia 22902 USA (1984). Obtainable from Oxford Psychologists Press (as above). (The ideas in this book on developing type were particularly useful for Chapter 12.)

Page, Earle. *Looking at Type*. Centre for Application of Psychological Type Inc., Florida, US (1983).